MORTAL EVIDENCE

MORTAL
The Forensics behind Nine Shocking Cases
EVIDENCE

CYRIL WECHT, M.D., J.D.
AND
GREG SAITZ
WITH
MARK CURRIDEN

FOREWORD BY DR. HENRY C. LEE

Prometheus Books

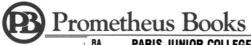

Published 2003 by Prometheus Books

Inquiries should be addressed to
Prometheus Books
59 John Glenn Drive
Amherst, New York 14228–2197
VOICE: 716–691–0133, ext. 207
FAX: 716–564–2711
WWW.PROMETHEUSBOOKS.COM

07 06 05 04 03   5 4 3 2 1

Library of Congress Cataloging-in-Publication Data

Wecht, Cyril H., 1931–
    Mortal evidence : the forensics behind nine shocking cases / Cyril Wecht and Greg Saitz, with Mark Curriden.
        p. cm.
    Includes bibliographical references (p.   ) and index.
    ISBN 1–59102–134–0 (alk. paper)
    1. Forensic pathology—Case studes. 2. Death—Causes—Case studies.
3. Criminal investigation—Case studies. I. Saitz, Greg. II. Curriden, Mark. III. Title.

RA1063.4.W433 2003
614'.1—dc22

                                                            2003016867

Printed in the United States of America on acid-free paper

CONTENTS

CONTENTS

FOREWORD

I FIRST MET CYRIL WECHT IN the early 1970s through the American Academy of Forensic Sciences. I was fairly new to the field, but Cyril already was well established as a major figure in forensic pathology. In the three decades since then, he has only added to his stature as one of the most astute medicolegal investigators in the world.

Over the years that we've known each other, we have given seminars and lectures together, and worked on many of the same cases. Sometimes, as you will read about in the O. J. Simpson case, we are on the same side. Other times we evaluate cases and come to different conclusions. But at the end of the day, even if we don't agree, we always respect one another's opinions.

In reaching those opinions, we often travel different roads. As a forensic scientist, I look at a crime scene and physical evidence such as blood spatters or fingerprints. In his role as a forensic pathologist, Cyril considers those things, but he focuses on a body—both inside and out—for critical clues. As you'll read in the case dealing with the death of Amy Grossberg and Brian Peterson's baby, the deductions that Cyril offers break away from those of the crowd.

And if there's one thing I've learned about Cyril, it's that he doesn't shy away from challenging the accepted line of thought. He speaks his mind, whether it diverges from the popular opinion or not. I believe everyone benefits when a person like Cyril dares to say that the emperor has no clothes.

In the case of JonBenet Ramsey, Cyril was one of the first, as you will read, to raise questions about the extent and timing of sexual abuse that the little girl endured before her death. He was largely attacked for voicing such an opinion. Although some other experts may disagree, we all respect his opinions.

Much of Cyril's sharpness comes from knowledge gained during an enviable career that spans more than four decades. While many who have reached his level of achievement and prominence delegate their workload, Cyril doggedly continues to pursue a dizzying array of investigations. He still conducts autopsies and actively works on cases both with the Allegheny County coroner's office and through consultations around the nation and the world.

And while I joke with Cyril that he has yet to learn how to send an e-mail, he continually updates his knowledge about the latest advances in the field of forensics, whether it be DNA testing or special histochemical stains. Such depth serves Cyril well, whether he is working in unraveling the details of the murder of Sam Sheppard's wife or explaining how the forensics tell a different story about a shoot-out in Arizona than was given by some authorities.

Taken as a whole, the cases Cyril recounts with flair in this book are not only informative, but also entertaining, illuminating, and thought provoking. And as always, Cyril doesn't pull any punches.

Dr. Henry C. Lee
Chief Emeritus for Scientific Services and
former Commissioner of Public Safety, State of Connecticut

PREFACE

OR MOST PEOPLE, death is an ending. For forensic pathologists, it's only a beginning. Like generations before us, we scientists are driven by the desire to understand how someone met his fate. Was it through natural causes or something more sinister?

Most deaths are easily categorized. About three-quarters of them are the result of old age or illness. Accidents make up the next largest group of the other quarter, followed by homicides and suicides. Finally, there are a small number of deaths whose cause is never determined. Despite great advances in medical and scientific technology, sometimes we still can't know for certain.

But more often than not, a body provides clues that can help solve the mystery of not only how that person died, but also how long ago, and in some cases of murder, by whose hand. "Pinpoint bleeding" on the inside of an individual's lower eyelids can be a sign of strangulation. Frothy fluid in the lungs may suggest a drug overdose death in a young adult who shows no signs of heart disease. Those details are critical to a forensic pathologist as he tries to determine the circumstances surrounding a death. After all, the field of forensic pathology is focused on delving into deaths that are violent, suspicious, sudden, unexplained, unexpected, or medically unattended.

Much attention is paid to deaths that are violent or suspicious—which is the realm of homicide detectives, criminalists, coroners, and medical examiners. All of those professions use forensic science to one degree or another to help solve cases. It can be a powerful tool; moreover, advances in the field have allowed practitioners to tease more clues out of less evidence. Forensic pathologists—coroners and medical examiners—are the ones who tie it all together. They perform the autopsy, collect information from the other investigators, analyze it, and make a conclusion about the cause and manner of death. That is my profession.

As forensic science has evolved, it increasingly has captured the interest of the public. All one has to do is look to prime-time television: *CSI: Crime Scene Investigation* and *CSI: Miami*, for instance, have emerged as two of the most watched programs in recent years. The shows have taken *Quincy* to a whole new level. Cable channels regularly feature shows such as *Cold Case Files*, *The New Detectives*, and *Medical Detectives* that frequently focus on cases solved by forensics. I have also noticed the public's fascination with such mysteries during the talks and seminars I give around the nation.

It's no wonder. The power of forensic science can help solve cases that otherwise would defy a solution as well as an explanation. One man's suspicious death was solved, as I describe in this book, by examining a few strands of hair. At the same time, forensics can help expose the reasons why someone has been wrongly accused of a crime. It's likely that some cases would have turned out differently if the available science and technology had been used in a timely fashion. Take the infamous murder of Dr. Sam Sheppard's wife in 1954. Had police and others who investigated the case used all the forensic tools at hand even then, I believe there's a good chance they would have excluded Dr. Sheppard early on as a suspect.

If there is one thing I have learned in my more than forty years of experience, having performed more than 14,000 autopsies and reviewed, signed off on, or supervised another 35,000 examinations, it is this: things are not always as they seem. One should not rush to judgment based on immediate assumptions. I have found that to be true in some of the most intensely scrutinized cases, including the assassinations of John F. Kennedy and his brother, Robert F. Kennedy, as well as ones that garner little, if any, attention.

In 1972 I was the first nongovernment forensic pathologist permitted to study the autopsy materials of President Kennedy, which had been preserved at the National Archives. Five years later, I was appointed to a nine-person forensic pathology panel established by the U.S. House Select Committee on Assassinations. Based on the evidence I reviewed at the National Archives, as well as other medical and forensic facts culled while on the panel and elsewhere, I concluded that the Warren Commission's single-bullet theory just couldn't be true. There was no way one bullet caused the wounds to Kennedy and Texas governor John Connally—who on November 22, 1963, was in the same motorcade with the president in Dallas.

Likewise, the June 1968 assassination of Sen. Robert Kennedy ultimately was attributed to one gunman—Sirhan Sirhan. But the forensic evidence suggested otherwise. Witnesses swore that Sirhan never got any closer than at least two feet from Kennedy during the incident. Yet forensics proved the fatal gunshot wound to Kennedy's head was fired at a much closer range—one to two inches from his skull. The evidence was soot blown from the gun's barrel that was found in Kennedy's hair and the wound. Additionally, there were characteristic markings of "stippling" on the senator's right ear, a sort of tattoo caused by burning gunpowder that is discharged from the gun's barrel. Those findings are seen only when a gun is fired at *very* close range.

But not every aspect of forensic pathology allows for such concrete conclusions. In fact, that applies to all divisions of medicine. Although many people mistakenly believe otherwise, medicine is not an absolute science. It's not physics or chemistry or mathematics. You can't take x plus y and always get the same result in medicine, because there is a significant subjective component in the analysis. That's often why patients are urged to get a second, or even a third, opinion regarding their medical diagnosis. Granted, pathology is on the least subjective end of a medical spectrum, with psychiatry at the opposite end. We pathologists get to hold tissues in our hands, measure, weigh, touch, smell, and look at evidence under the microscope.

Still, differences of opinions can and do occur. To understand that, all one has to do is attend conferences where pathologists gather to discuss difficult and complex cases. Usually, slides and other medical information are sent to participants in advance, and then a moderator running the conference will ask the pathologists for their opinions. It's not uncommon in a room of thirty or forty board-certified pathologists to have them come up with three, four, or even five varying diagnoses.

If the question is what does a particular patient have on her leg, one doctor might say it's an atypical variant of a benign tumor and recommend that nothing more need be done than excise it locally and observe it thereafter periodically. Another equally qualified pathologist may believe that the tumor is malignant and the patient should have her leg amputated at the hip to keep it from spreading and to save her life. I've been at some conferences where the participants become so engaged and passionate about their positions they stop just short of fisticuffs. While such behavior certainly isn't socially acceptable, it's an extreme form of what is considered good, academic, freewheeling discussion and debate among educated professionals.

However, take that disagreement out of the context of a scholarly conference, where the matter of who's right and who's wrong is to some degree a matter of pride, and place it instead in a courtroom in a medical malpractice case or a criminal trial, and the stakes are much higher. All of a sudden, a difference of opinions expressed by two medical experts takes on new meaning. Moreover, many believe that doctors who consult with attorneys and testify in court are acting as medical prostitutes, providing testimony for money. That to me is intellectual nonsense and hypocrisy in its most basic form.

For the past four decades, I have offered testimony in courtrooms around the country in civil cases ranging from personal injury to medical malpractice to product liability. On the criminal side, I have consulted with defense attorneys and prosecutors alike, sometimes even with the U.S. Department of Justice. I also am called upon to testify in and around Pittsburgh as the elected coroner of Allegheny County. In every instance, my findings have been based on the medical and forensic evidence. To do otherwise would be unthinkable.

I have played a role in every case recounted here within the criminal and/or civil justice system with the exception of the Jon-Benet Ramsey case. For that, I have been and continue to act as a commentator for CNN and other television networks.

As forensic scientific technology and expertise continue to advance, both the civil and the criminal justice systems will benefit significantly in their ability to provide just verdicts. Law school professors Barry Scheck and Peter Neufeld, through the Innocence Project they established in 1992, have used DNA evidence to prove that more than 130 individuals convicted of various crimes, including murder, were innocent. I intend to continue using the latest forensic advances to work toward obtaining the truth in criminal and civil cases.

I hope that through these pages readers will better understand the interrelationship of science and law and appreciate the benefits that accrue to society by such a professional marriage. I have tried to make the chapters informative and illuminating, as well as accessible. Enjoy the journey.

Cyril Wecht, M.D., J.D.

ACKNOWLEDGMENTS

THERE ARE MANY PEOPLE TO THANK for helping us with this book from its earliest stages to the final manuscript. Words of encouragement, words of advice, and words of wisdom all were welcomed.

For their overall contributions, we would like to thank Drs. Michael Baden and Henry C. Lee. Attorney Terry Gilbert, who was dedicated to revealing the truth in the Sam Sheppard case, was more than gracious with his time, insight, and files. Judge Peter Paul Olszewski Jr., former district attorney for Luzerne County, Pennsylvania, also took time from his schedule to provide assistance with the Robert Curley case.

For their assistance with the Miracle Valley chapter, we would like to thank Arizona attorney Armond Salese and Bud Foster, a television reporter. The chapter on JonBenet Ramsey

ACKNOWLEDGMENTS

would have been impossible without the initial hard work of Charles Bosworth Jr.

At Prometheus Books, our editor, Linda Greenspan Regan, helped us focus and refine the project, and we thank her for her efforts. Michaela Hamilton deserves thanks for her early contributions and guidance. At the Allegheny County coroner's office, Kathy McCabe and Eileen Young helped us keep organized and on track. Jaki Hathcock helped by transcribing tapes and researching old newspaper articles.

Finally, none of this would have been possible without the support of our families.

Chapter One

TEENAGE BABY KILLERS?

The Truth behind the Death of Baby Boy Grossberg

ON NOVEMBER 12, 1996, AMY GROSSBERG and Brian Peterson were just two anonymous college freshmen, two teenagers with promising futures from upper-middle-class homes in northern New Jersey. Eighteen-year-old Grossberg, in her first semester at the University of Delaware, was a pretty brunette who liked art. Peterson, her boyfriend since high school, was handsome and athletic and attending Gettysburg College in Pennsylvania. But less than a week later, they were the talk of the nation, and much of the world—branded as heartless baby killers. They also were the subjects of an aggressive team of prosecutors seeking a murder conviction and a death sentence.

Eventually, what happened in room 220 of the Comfort Inn in Newark, Delaware, was debated not only by those involved in the criminal case, but also by newspaper columnists, television talk-show hosts, and millions of everyday citizens. Were Grossberg and Peterson two unfeeling animals who, after delivering their infant son in the hotel, viciously murdered him and tossed his tiny body into a nearby Dumpster? Or were they scared and confused young people who panicked after Grossberg gave birth to a blue and seemingly lifeless baby?

The questions touched a nerve with so many people because it was easy for them to imagine Grossberg and Peterson as their daughter, their son, their neighbors, or maybe even themselves. Grossberg grew up in Wyckoff and Franklin Lakes, New Jersey, two leafy and affluent neighborhoods in the northeast corner of the state. Her parents, Alan and Sonye, owned a furniture business and worked hard to achieve their success. Peterson spent much of his youth on Long Island before moving to Wyckoff to live with his mother, Barbara Zuchowski, and stepfather, John, who together ran a video wholesale company. The two teenagers met at Ramapo High School, where Peterson was the soccer cocaptain, and they started dating in their sophomore year. They continued to see each other during their first semester of college, which was cut short by their arrests.

Almost immediately, a debate erupted over whether authorities should pursue premeditated, first-degree murder charges against Amy and Brian. But there also was a less well-known debate over the medical issues. Once I consulted with Grossberg's defense team and had a chance to review the available evidence in the case, I was shocked on two levels. One was the single-minded intensity with which authorities pursued their case. The other was the pathological evidence that clearly indicated to me, and several other medical experts, that the baby either was stillborn or died shortly after birth; he had severe congenital problems that made his survival impossible.

Initially, I learned of the case through the media. I read the *New York Times* every day, and there was a story in its November 18,

1996, edition. Two days earlier, on Saturday, authorities issued first-degree murder warrants for Grossberg and Peterson. Investigators became involved the evening of November 12, after Grossberg suffered seizures and began bleeding on campus and was rushed to the hospital. Medical personnel discovered the undelivered placenta and diagnosed Grossberg as suffering from eclampsia, a serious illness brought on by childbirth that affects not only the mother, but also the baby. However, the baby was nowhere to be found, and hospital workers contacted police. Officers then went to speak with Peterson, who told them he and Grossberg had "gotten rid of the baby." A search dog found the baby's body in the Dumpster about twenty-four hours after Peterson had put it there.

The *Times* story quoted from an autopsy report, which determined the infant's cause of death to be "multiple fractures (linear and depressed) with injury to the brain due to blunt force head trauma and shaking." The article also quoted a deputy attorney general saying prosecutors would seek the death penalty. And later that night, Delaware attorney general M. Jane Brady was live via phone on Geraldo Rivera's cable television show, *Rivera Live*: "Based on the information we have and the autopsy results, we believe that the injuries were intentionally inflicted, and in our state, . . . those acts constitute murder in the first degree."

I was absolutely stunned at the state's approach. Just five days had passed since investigators found the baby and conducted an autopsy. That was not nearly enough time for them to have completed a thorough investigation by any means, much less to have gotten critical input from other medical specialists such as a neuropathologist. Yet prosecutors seemed to be telling anyone who would listen that they had a clear case of premeditated, first-degree murder.

It is unfortunate, but cases such as these happen more often than anyone would like to imagine. An unwed teenage mother who has hidden her pregnancy from her parents and everyone else gives birth, and through either some sort of neglect or a more intentional act, the baby dies. There's no question the mother or both parents should be held accountable in some way. But first-degree murder, with the penalties upon conviction being at least life in prison, if not the death penalty?

The representatives of the state's case seemed excessive in their statements and premature judgments. I believe that everything in life is relative, including the administration of justice and penalties. So if officials for the state of Delaware were calling what happened with Grossberg and Peterson first-degree murder, what would they call a case of a serial killer, or someone who deliberately rapes and murders a ten-year-old girl? Those crimes certainly seem more heinous and I think most people would agree deserving of a harsher punishment than two teenagers who, once the facts were in, clearly did not commit first-degree murder. At any rate, how does a system penalize more hardened and heinous criminals *more* than what prosecutors said they wanted to do to Grossberg and Peterson? Do you torture the child rapist and murderer before executing him? Not according to the Constitution. Sure, the argument becomes absurd, but it gets to my point: the authorities really seemed to have rushed to judgment too quickly and much too forcefully in this case.

In other countries—including Great Britain, from which the United States derives its form of common law—infanticide is considered separate and distinct from other murder charges. A subcategory of neonaticide refers to deaths within the first thirty days of birth. If a mother is accused of killing her child who is less than a year old and "the balance of her mind was disturbed by having given birth," the maximum charge she can face is manslaughter.[1] In fact, a psychological condition that affects some new mothers, known as postpartum depression, is an applicable legal defense in twenty-nine countries. Those countries, which include Canada, Australia, and Italy, realize the unique and often dire circumstances

22

women may find themselves in when it comes to their newborn or infant children.

In any case, I was glad to see that Harvard law professor Alan Dershowitz, who also was on Geraldo's show, shared my opinion. He challenged the attorney general's position that Grossberg and Peterson should face capital murder charges. "There are 3,500 people on death row for more than 100,000 murders. You just don't charge a mother with first-degree murder and capital punishment for the post-traumatic birth syndrome killing of a child," Dershowitz said. "It's tragically common that people get very depressed after they give birth, and it's just unheard of in a civilized society to charge a woman with murder for this."[2]

* • •

I kept an eye on the case as it progressed. The day the *Times* story appeared, officers arrested Grossberg after she was released from Christiana Hospital in Delaware. Peterson remained at large for several more days, but eventually turned himself in at the FBI offices in Wilmington, Delaware. He had been with his parents and stepfather at a hotel in the city while his attorney, Joseph Hurley, talked with authorities about the teenager's surrender. (Officials had declared Peterson a fugitive and issued a federal arrest warrant for him.) His arrival at the building that housed the FBI was not a secret. Hurley had told the media about it, and hundreds of reporters and television camera crews were waiting. Peterson, wearing a ball cap and a fleece jacket, was flanked by his parents, and as they pushed through the crowd, FBI agents rushed outside to shepherd them through the gauntlet. Someone in the crowd yelled out, "Baby killer!"

Once inside the building, Peterson and his mother both cried, according to Hurley. Now that Peterson had surrendered, Hurley addressed the media throng that had taken such an interest in the case. He acknowledged that Peterson had used bad judgment but said that what happened wasn't murder. "He did something wrong," Hurley said. "But we're not sure what he did wrong." At a court hearing later that day, Peterson was ordered held without bail, the same as Grossberg.

In the first week after Grossberg and Peterson were arrested, defense attorneys raised the possibility that the baby was stillborn, a reasonable theory given Peterson's description of the infant upon birth—blue and lifeless. The Delaware medical examiner's office tried to knock down any suggestion of the sort. Officials said the baby was a full-term, healthy boy who was born alive and showed no signs of birth defects or deformities.[3]

For the Thanksgiving week that year, which began just a few days after the arrests of Grossberg and Peterson, I was able to get away on a short family vacation. If possible, I always like to go somewhere with my wife, my grown children, and their families for the holiday. This time we went to Florida. While there, I learned Hurley wanted to get in touch with me. I contacted him and eventually had a phone conference with Hurley and Dr. Michael Baden, who the defense already had retained. Dr. Baden, who is a close personal friend, is one of the top forensic pathologists in the country and the former chief medical examiner of New York City. "I think we're going to have to get a forensic neuropathologist and an expert in high-risk obstetrics," I said. The neuropathologist would conduct a through and detailed examination of the baby's brain and an obstetrics expert would review Grossberg's clinical scenario before, during, and after delivery.

I was scheduled to fly to Delaware that Monday to join Dr. Baden in an examination of the baby's body, but there was a last-minute change and I never made the trip. From what I understood, another attorney hired to help defend Peterson decided another forensic pathologist was not needed at that point on the case.

Although I was puzzled by the decision, I nonetheless told Hurley to contact me if they wanted my assistance in the future.

Several months passed and I didn't hear from anyone involved in the case. However, I continued to read about the latest developments. A grand jury indicted Grossberg and Peterson in December on charges of first-degree murder. On December 17, the two appeared in court to enter not guilty pleas. It was the first time they had seen each other since before their arrests. Grossberg was being held at the Dolores J. Baylor Women's Correctional Institution in New Castle, Delaware, while Peterson was detained at Gander Hill Prison in Wilmington. Superior Court Judge Henry duPont Ridgely refused to grant the teenagers bail but said he would reconsider the issue at another hearing in January.

At that hearing, held January 21, Judge Ridgely agreed to release the couple on $300,000 bail each. But there were conditions: they had to relinquish their passports, sign extradition waivers, live with their parents, and wear electronic monitoring devices attached to their ankles. They also were required to comply with an 8 P.M. to 6 A.M. curfew. Grossberg and Peterson were released later that day, but did not return to New Jersey until January 31, after a monitoring system had been set in place. Once again, the news helicopters hovered and crowds of reporters clogged the streets near the college freshmen's homes about a mile apart from each other. Peterson, his mother, and one of his attorneys, Russell Gioiella, came out of the house briefly, but Peterson did not speak. "I hope you all will give him a chance to be with his family in the privacy of their home," Gioiella said to the mass of reporters.[4]

Then in late May 1997, I received a call from Robert Gottlieb, one of Grossberg's new attorneys. He asked if I would consult on the case to help determine whether the baby was born alive and whether there were any injuries he sustained during birth or any congenital anomalies that would have made his survival implausible. I again agreed, and this time there were no last-minute changes.

By then, several other highly qualified medical experts already were consulting with attorneys for Grossberg and Peterson. Michael Baden, of course, still was involved. The team also consisted of Dr. Harlan Giles, a specialist in obstetrics and gynecology from Pittsburgh with extensive experience in genetics, prenatal diagnosis, and birth defects; Dr. Jan Leestma, considered the top forensic neuropathologist in the country and probably the world; and Dr. Janice Ophoven, a nationally known pediatric forensic pathologist.

The next day, I received from Gottlieb a thick packet of documents that included the autopsy report and associated notes, reports from experts whom prosecutors had consulted, copies of slides from the baby's brain dissection, and other correspondence. While I had read and heard media accounts of what the medical examiner claimed to have found during the autopsy, I was eager to see first-hand the medical reports that the authorities were relying on to support a charge of first-degree murder.

Conducting autopsies on newborns and other children is not technically difficult. It is important to document every injury, get adequate x-rays, and perform all the other normal procedures associated with a postmortem examination. But emotionally, it's a different story. Of the thousands of autopsies I've done during the past forty-six years, probably a couple of hundred of them have been on infants and maybe a couple of dozen were on abandoned newborns. I find those cases always more emotionally charged and viscerally disturbing than similar ones involving adults.

I'm not saying that I am insensitive to the brutal deaths of adults, but those of infants or young children make me realize the vulnerability of innocence and the fragility of life. A child has little if any ability to defend himself or herself. And unquestionably absent is any deliberate action on the young victim's part to provoke the horrible crime committed against him or her. They had no say in the way their lives ended, and now they won't have a chance to grow and become a thriving, productive human being.

However, I try very hard not to let the emotional aspect of such cases interfere with my job of determining what may have happened. While the death of any newborn is tragic, it's not always criminal. Sometimes natural deliveries can cause unusual head trauma, and that can be difficult to differentiate from a deliberately inflicted injury. The same goes for resolving whether a baby was born alive. It's not always an easy and clear-cut determination, and I soon realized such an analysis would most likely prove to be quite difficult in this case.

When the infant's body arrived at the Delaware medical examiner's office the morning of November 13, 1996, assistant medical examiner Dr. Adrienne Sekula-Perlman noted it was cold to the touch. She described the baby, called "Baby Boy Grossberg," as "normally developed" and weighing 6.2 pounds. However, small amounts of meconium—intestinal content that comes out of a baby through its anal opening in utero—were noted on the legs and buttocks. That's not an ordinary finding, and to me it was evidence the baby was in distress in Grossberg's womb, which caused the meconium to be expelled.

Perlman found no abrasions or lacerations on the face, head, or body. She also did not find any bone or rib fractures and saw no evidence of injury prior to shaving the hair on the infant's head. After that, Perlman noted multiple skull fractures and described extensive hemorrhaging. There was a well-defined purple-red bruise on the top of the head. One fracture was on the top of the head, another generally to the left and a third more to the right. Upon removing the skull, Perlman described finding an epidural hemorrhage.

To understand where these are, it helps to visualize several different layers between the actual brain and the skull. The first layer over the brain is called pia mater, which essentially is the outermost layer of brain cells and can't be seen with the naked eye. After that comes the arachnoid, named so because it has a delicate pattern similar to a spider web, followed by the dura, a thicker and tougher opaque membrane just below the skull. To locate certain findings, medical examiners and pathologists refer to them as being either epi—outside—or sub—meaning below. So an epidural hemorrhage is one found outside the dura membrane. Perlman also described subdural hemorrhages as well as areas that appeared to her to be consistent with subarachnoid hemorrhages. The eyes showed retinal hemorrhages.

Internally, she found the body cavities free of blood and the organs in the correct positions. "There are no gross abnormalities noted which are incompatible with life," Perlman wrote. She described both lungs as "well expanded" and said she found air in the gastrointestinal tract. Perlman also submerged sections of the lungs in liquid and they floated. The technique, used since medieval times, is pretty basic. If the lungs float, that means they contain air, and if they have air that means the baby breathed. But the method is simplistic and not always accurate. It should be used in conjunction with other tests and observations—particularly under the microscope—to make a valid determination as to whether a newborn took in air. Additionally, according to Perlman, x-rays showed air in the lungs and in the small intestines.

Perlman listed the cause of death as "multiple skull fractures (linear and depressed) with epidural, subdural, and subarachnoid hemorrhages, hypothermia and asphyxia." So she was saying, in essence, that not only did the head trauma contribute to the baby's death, but what also played a part was the cold temperature the infant was exposed to in the Dumpster and a lack of oxygen from being sealed in a gray plastic trash bag. As a secondary cause of death in her final autopsy report released many months later, Perlman listed schizencephaly.

Schizencephaly is a rare and severe congenital brain malformation. It is essentially a cleft in the brain, a separation of brain tissue. This abnormality can lead to a stillbirth. In the event the baby is born alive, he or she would have major physiological problems such as cerebral palsy and likely would not survive for more than a year. That wasn't a finding authorities seemed eager to disseminate. In fact, I noticed prosecutors didn't release the full autopsy report (with the schizencephaly finding) to defense attorneys until the spring of 1997, many months after the November 1996 autopsy. To be fair, the neuropathological examination and microscopic sectioning of the brain was performed December 13, 1996, but only after defense attorneys requested that it be done. Dr. Lucy Rorke, a neuropathologist from Philadelphia, performed the sectioning for the state in the presence of Drs. Baden and Leestma, and that was when the brain defects were noted. But by then, the public's perception of what had happened had already had been fixed by the original comments made by authorities: that the baby died of head trauma, asphyxia, and hypothermia.

●　●　●

Soon after I joined the case, Amy Grossberg, her parents, and Gottlieb appeared in early June 1997 on the television news program *20/20*. The night the show aired, June 6, another case of a young mother accused of killing her baby was just beginning. Melissa Drexler, an eighteen-year-old high-school senior in central New Jersey, gave birth in a bathroom at her prom that evening, allegedly strangled her baby, and threw him away. She eventually was charged with murder, but the prosecutor in that case declined to seek the death penalty. He told reporters that he considered the mental strain Drexler was under at the time of birth. "It's hard to justify any of this, but we're talking about emotional conduct, someone who isn't thinking clearly," Monmouth County prosecutor John Kaye said. "It's generally not knowing, purposeful murder. These cases are usually resolved with a manslaughter charge."[5]

For Amy and her parents, the TV program would be the first time they spoke publicly about the case, and they did so despite a gag order imposed by the presiding judge on many of those involved. Host Barbara Walters first interviewed Sonye and Alan Grossberg, who tried to dispel the perceptions that they were the privileged elite and their daughter was some sort of monster. Her parents said that they never suspected Amy was pregnant, attributing a slight weight gain they had noticed two weeks before the birth to the "freshman fifteen" pounds that girls sometimes put on when they go away to college.

"Your daughter has been described as a baby killer," Walters said. "What do you most want people to know about Amy?"

"I want people to know, number one, she wouldn't hurt her baby, anybody's baby," Sonye Grossberg replied. "She's always so giving and caring. I can't believe that people don't see that about her."

Later in the program, Amy spoke with Walters. Grossberg said she had always had irregular periods and wasn't particularly worried about missing one. She also recounted the night she was rushed to the hospital with seizures, and what it was like to be accused of first-degree murder and face the death penalty.

"Have you been to the cemetery to visit the baby's grave?" Walters asked.

"Yes, I have," Amy said.

"Do you mourn the loss of that baby?"

"Of course," Grossberg said. "It was part of me. My heart breaks. I would never hurt anything or anybody, especially something that could come from me."

For his participation in the show—as minimal as it was—Gottlieb was removed from the case by the judge at the urging of prosecutors.

●　•　●

Listening to Amy and her parents on TV was one thing, but I felt talking to her directly about what she remembered and how events progressed would be much more helpful to my work on the case. We met in Philadelphia in mid-November at the home of another of Grossberg's attorneys, Jack Gruenstein. By then, the Grossbergs had replaced Gottlieb with Beverly Hills attorney Bob Tanenbaum, whom I knew quite well from previous work. Tanenbaum is a well-known author and highly experienced trial attorney, who once had been the chief homicide prosecutor in the Manhattan District Attorney's Office. Michael Baden also was there.

Amy was pleasant and didn't seem like she was trying to impress anyone. She struck me as a scared young woman who had been through a great deal. Fortunately for her, I also noticed, she had strong support from her parents. She told us about the summer of 1996, which she spent as a camp counselor, and of a July 1996 physical that had been given by her doctor. During the exam, her internist never noted her pregnancy, despite the fact she was about five months along at that point. Amy said she was unaware as well.

Amy told us what she could remember about the delivery and the events leading up to it. By the time she and Peterson arrived at the motel, she knew that she was pregnant. She recalled lying in the bed at the motel, then feeling pressure and something surge out of her. But she said her eyes were closed and she wasn't really aware of what was happening. I wasn't surprised, given that from what we knew, Amy had been suffering from preeclampsia, a condition that affects some pregnant women. Mainly, it causes a woman's blood pressure to rise—a pregnancy-induced hypertension—and, in Amy's case, it manifested itself days before the birth. If it is not dealt with, the condition can progress to eclampsia, a much more serious and life-threatening situation.

Dr. Carol Tavani is a psychiatrist and chief of staff at Christiana Hospital, where Amy was taken suffering from seizures fourteen hours after the delivery. Tavani talked with Amy at the hospital and, based on the symptoms Amy described, Tavani later concluded that Amy was in a state of preeclampsia as early as November 9, 1996, three days before giving birth. Those signs included worsening epigastric pain that progressed to vomiting, increased lethargy, blurred vision, and light sensitivity, which eventually progressed to a deterioration of cognitive clarity. In short, Amy was in a fog. She obviously wasn't thinking straight; thus it was illogical to me that she should be expected to totally comprehend what was happening and respond properly.

Amy's state of preeclampsia and eventual eclampsia also played an important role in terms of how it affected the baby. Those conditions are stressful not just to the mother, but also to the infant, which fit in with the other medical evidence that I had examined before the meeting with Amy and her parents.

Drs. Giles and Ophoven and I looked at tissue samples and portions of the infant's brain at the Delaware medical examiner's office. Later, after reviewing other tissue slides at my office, Dr. Baden and I flew to Chicago to discuss the importance of the various findings with Dr. Leestma. We had a lot to talk about. One issue involved the nerve cells of the infant's brain, the neurons. As with other cells in the body, brain cells that are deprived of oxygen die. Those dead brain cells can later be differentiated from other cells because they shrink and give off a red appearance. Pathologists call them red dead neurons. Slides of the baby's brain showed red neurons all over the place.

But the changes don't manifest themselves right away. It usually takes one and a half to two hours after the oxygen-depriving incident—referred to as an insult to the brain—for cells to begin transforming. And it's not until between four and eight hours later that these changes can be observed. The catch is the baby has to be "alive" for those changes to occur. Therefore, that finding would have seemed to support the medical examiner's contention of a viable birth. However, the definition of alive includes intrauterine life—the time that the infant was still in Grossberg's womb. In addition, Drs. Leestma and Baden and I discussed four compelling reasons why the baby was likely either stillborn or lived only briefly after birth.

1. There was no vital reaction in the baby's lungs or elsewhere in the body. A vital reaction is an early inflammatory response and takes several minutes to develop. It won't happen with one or two breaths. Whenever tissues are damaged for whatever reason—from a virus or bacteria, or maybe too much heat or cold—white blood cells in the body rush to the scene to act as soldiers of defense. That response can usually be seen under the microscope within an hour or two. But in this case, the slides didn't show that.
2. There was no brain swelling. Simply put, when a person, even a baby, is alive and the brain is deprived of oxygen, it will swell.
3. There was no real expansion of the tiny air sacs in the lungs called alveoli. The lungs contain hundreds of thousands of alveoli, and if air is breathed in, these alveoli will expand. When the air sacs aren't expanded, however, they lay flat atop each other, layer upon layer. Dr. Perlman, the assistant medical examiner, wrote in the autopsy report: "Good expansion of the lungs is evidenced by widespread irregu-

33

larly expanded alveoli throughout . . ." I looked at the same microscopic slides that Dr. Perlman did. So did Dr. Leestma and the other medical experts working with the defense. None of us saw widespread irregularly expanded alveoli.

4. There was no evidence of hemorrhaging at the fracture sites of the skull. Dr. Perlman devoted a good amount of space in the autopsy report describing the skull fractures and associated hemorrhages. She noted blood along the fracture lines, but such a finding wasn't visible in the photographs taken of the fractures. And that is key, because if a fracture occurs when someone is alive, there will be some bleeding. Bone is a spongy tissue, and a fractured bone will soak up some blood along the fracture line, leaving a clear indication as to whether it occurred before or after death. Also, had the fractures occurred when the baby was alive, there would have been massive bleeding, and that wasn't found by any of us.

After establishing those four particulars, we went back to the red neuron finding. We know several hours must pass with the infant being "alive" for these red neurons to form. But a lack of vital reaction in the tissues in addition to the other signs clearly showed that the baby could not have survived for that long after birth. The changes to the brain therefore had to have occurred while the infant was still in Grossberg's uterus.

The cause of the red neurons was the stress that the baby was subjected to in utero. There were other signs of strain on the infant, too, and they all conspired to affect his health. One was the meconium that stained his body and the placental tissues. It was more extensive than noted in the autopsy. Though Dr. Perlman did not note meconium staining on the baby's fingernail beds, Dr. Ophoven did while reviewing photographs of the body. Another indication of stress was the condition of the placenta. The surface of a placenta has tiny projections on it called villi. In a normal placenta, one would expect to find about 30 percent of the villi knotted. Here, nearly all of them were, which denotes stress in utero, or inside the womb. So what caused the stress? A major contributing factor was Grossberg's preeclamptic and eclamptic condition, which would have cut down dramatically on how much oxygen and blood the baby received from the placenta.

Moreover, that lack of oxygen and blood flow in the hours just prior to the baby's birth caused irreversible brain damage. And this was in addition to the considerable congenital anomalies already present in the brain. Further examination of the brain showed not only the schizencephaly, but also a host of other rare and disabling abnormalities. Coinciding with the schizencephaly was a large porencephalic cyst, an opening caused by a loss of brain tissue that is instead filled with fluid. Sections of the brain examined under the microscope revealed other problems. There were signs of poly-microgyria—abnormal cells—in several areas, as well as hetero-topias, tissues of the brain found in the wrong place. The slides also revealed hypogenesis (inadequate development) of the corti-cospinal tract, a very important nerve component that comes down from the brain into the spinal cord. Furthermore, in the part of the brain where the spinal fluid is formed were multiple areas of dead cells and calcification. Lastly, multiple areas throughout the gray matter of the brain showed gliosis, that is, scarring, which can impair the infant's ability to move both inside the womb and after birth. These were all *developmental defects* entirely unconnected to any head trauma.

So it's entirely logical to believe that when this infant was born, it appeared still and lifeless, as Peterson had described. He said that it came out spontaneously, face down, blue, and limp. But despite the baby's appearance, not to mention its neurological devastation, there still remained the question of whether he was born alive. I have my doubts, and the severe distress that the baby experienced in utero seems to support a stillbirth. However, x-rays of the intestines showed air or gas in the gut. After discussing this with other defense medical experts, I concluded that it meant one of two things. The first possibility was the infant, through an involuntary movement, took what is called an agonal gasp or two in an attempt to get air. It by no means is evidence of a healthy live child. Based on what we knew about the baby, it could not have lived outside the uterus for more than a few minutes. As Drs. Leestma and Ophoven noted at one point, even at the best hospital in the world the baby would have been considered brain dead and quite possibly could not have been resuscitated. The other plausible reason for gas in that area of the intestine would be from decomposition. Tissues in the body begin to decompose after death, and the rate of that breakdown depends on physical conditions of the environment. For example, the warmer it is, the more rapid the process. The bacteria that form can very quickly lead to the production of gasses, which can be misinterpreted as breathed-in air in the lungs. In this case, the infant was in the Dumpster for more than twenty-four hours before being recovered by police. That was more than enough time for postmortem decomposition to have begun and for gasses to have formed in the tissues, including the lungs. Such changes would be even more evident in an infant exposed to the elements, because the proportion of body surface to total body weight is greater in a baby as compared to an adult.

We also wanted to address the characterization by Dr. Perlman that the baby was "normal" in its physical appearance. To the contrary, we all noted that photos of the baby prior to the autopsy clearly showed an asymmetry. The baby's left arm was smaller than his right and the chest appeared sunken. There also was evidence that the left side of his body was paralyzed.

That left the head trauma, which the medical examiner concluded was caused by a purposeful act. The defense experts, myself included, thought the damage more likely occurred during delivery and subsequently, when the baby was put in the trash bin. It is not uncommon to see significant head trauma during a delivery where there are no skilled medical personnel in attendance and when a young girl with a small pelvis is delivering her first child. Sometimes, babies descend into the birth canal quickly and bang the tops of their heads on the mother's pelvis. The result can be hemorrhaging beneath the scalp, known as caput succadaneum. Even fracturing of the skull can occur in some instances.

The hemorrhaging in the Grossberg baby, including the retinal hemorrhages Dr. Perlman ascribed to shaking, could just as easily have been caused by an explosive, precipitous delivery. That is entirely consistent with Grossberg's recollection that she felt something squish out of her within an hour of arriving at the hotel. The bleeding was made worse by the position of the baby in the Dumpster for twenty-five hours; signs found at the autopsy indicated the infant's right side and head were lower in the Dumpster than other parts of his body, causing blood to pool there.

●　•　●

My conclusions and the conclusions of the other experts working for Grossberg and Peterson were presented to the prosecutors by defense attorneys toward the end of 1997. But authorities seemed adamant in their position. They had consulted with their own forensic pathology experts, who offered opinions supporting the medical examiner's diagnosis and downplaying the seriousness of the congenital brain defects. Even though it was acknowledged that the hemorrhages in the baby's eyes could have been caused from the unattended birth process, Dr. Perlman was resolute in her belief the head trauma was caused by a purposeful act.

As mentioned before, the death of a child, especially an infant, brings into play an emotional element that is not usually present in other cases. We've reached a point in the United States that when a child or infant is brought into a hospital with an injury, it is viewed as a case of likely or possible child abuse before it is ruled out. In other words, the burden is on the parents or guardian to prove whatever happened was an accident. That's not to say the injury, or even death, might have been the result of negligence in some way. Just as there are negligent and incompetent doctors in the world who shouldn't be practicing medicine, there are some people who shouldn't be parents. But to make such a huge leap from negligence—or "how could you be so stupid?"—to murder is a stretch.

Yet I believe too many of my colleagues in forensic pathology have succumbed to this way of approaching cases. They too readily accept what authorities may tell them about a case instead of letting the totality of the evidence lead them to form an objective conclusion. In this case, the conclusions of one of the state's experts, a competent forensic pathologist, were at odds with my opinions on almost every issue, as well as those of Drs. Leestma, Ophoven, and Baden. The prosecution's experts did not even consider our findings to have been possible, which would have created a reasonable doubt regarding Grossberg's murder charge.

The trial date, meanwhile, had been postponed from October 1997 to May 1998 to give Grossberg's new lawyers more time to prepare. All the while, news stories continued to appear, and one in particular caught my eye. The article in the *Record*, a New Jersey newspaper, examined the issue of whether parents should be forced to reveal conversations they've had with their children. Prosecutors in this case had subpoenaed Amy's parents in search of incriminating evidence. I sent copies to Drs. Baden, Giles, Leestma, and Ophoven with a small note: "It's truly incredible how the Delaware prosecutors have made this into the most horrendous crime ever committed in their jurisdiction. Small town mentality doesn't explain this phenomenon adequately."

As the months passed, the once-united front presented by Grossberg and Peterson began to disintegrate. In January 1998, Grossberg's attorneys asked the judge to give the two teenagers separate trials, noting that their defenses were incompatible. To believe her defense, jurors would have to reject his defense. After all, it was Peterson who told police early on that he got rid of the baby and threw it out. That was followed in early March by a court filing by Grossberg's attorneys, who said she passed two polygraph tests administered by her defense team in November 1997 regarding the birth at the motel. The motion requesting the results be admitted as evidence listed several questions and answers from the lie detector tests. In the answers, she denied that she and Peterson planned to kill the baby and said she believed that she had had a miscarriage.

Soon, however, the polygraph results were not the biggest development in the case, and what happened next made the issue of separate trials moot.

On March 9, Peterson walked into court with his parents and pleaded guilty to manslaughter. As part of the deal with prosecutors, he agreed to testify against his one-time girlfriend in her upcoming May trial. During the hearing, one of Peterson's attorneys explained to Judge Ridgely what happened that November morning.

"After the baby was born, the infant did not show any signs of life, and he believed the baby was dead," attorney Russell Gioiella said. "He acknowledges great regret that they did not summon medical aid. He did not confirm it was dead. Amy is telling Brian, 'Get rid of it, get rid of it,' and Brian eventually puts the baby in a bag and throws it in a Dumpster outside the motel."[6]

As a doctor, I question the extent to which Grossberg would have been mentally capable of ordering Peterson around. It's been a long time since I delivered babies—more than forty-five years ago during medical school and residency. But I remember some women were just out of it mentally during the final phase of delivery. In Amy's case, add the preeclampsia and eclampsia she was suffering from that would have diminished her cognitive abilities. I'm sure she wasn't thinking clearly, let alone having the intellectual ability to coordinate the disposal of her baby.

Six weeks after Peterson's court appearance, Grossberg arrived at the courthouse in Wilmington, Delaware. She was sobbing as she made her way inside. Bob Tanenbaum, a big, tall man, wrapped a protective arm around her shoulder, and her mother clutched her hand. In the courtroom before Judge Ridgely, Grossberg pleaded guilty to the same manslaughter charge Peterson had. Tanenbaum told the judge Grossberg was taking full responsibility for what happened, but that she never meant to hurt the baby and wasn't involved in discarding his body. One of the prosecutors countered that Grossberg showed a "chilling indifference" to the baby's life.

Sentencing for both Grossberg and Peterson came July 9. Each faced up to ten years in prison, but sentencing guidelines suggested a more lenient term of two and a half years. As they had throughout the case, prosecutors depicted Amy Grossberg as cold and calculating in her refusal to notify anyone about her pregnancy and in her attitude regarding the death of her baby. Deputy Attorney General Peter Letang read from letters she wrote to Peterson when they started college, one of which said, "All I want for it is to go away." For her part, Amy showed contrition. "I'm extremely sorry for what happened to my baby. I blame nobody but myself."

The judge listened, then chastised Grossberg for her failure to seek help before giving birth and sentenced her to two and a half years in prison, to be followed by probation and three hundred hours of community service. Peterson came next, but Ridgely imposed just a two-year sentence on him, noting the young man's cooperation with prosecutors and his efforts to have Grossberg get medical help for the delivery.

That was the end of the case. Both sides still disagreed about how the baby died. Still, the plea bargaining to significantly downgraded charges was an indication to me that the authorities knew they could not prove first-degree murder. In later comments, the prosecutor acknowledged problems in proving how the baby's head injuries occurred.

I don't take the position that Grossberg and Peterson should not have received some sort of punishment in this case. Her failure to go to a doctor or tell anyone about the pregnancy no doubt was wrong and negligent. Their decision to head to a motel room that fateful morning instead of a hospital also was not the right one. However, I don't believe it was made with any sort of forethought of the eventual consequences or for some nefarious purpose. I'm not even sure they knew where they were going when they left Grossberg's dorm. She was sick, scared, and panicked about the situation in which she found herself. Both she and Peterson had hidden her pregnancy from everyone, even their parents. Peterson was no doubt anxious as well and wanted to comfort his ailing girlfriend. But at that point, they must have believed they had only each other to turn to for guidance and support in a predicament very few teenagers are capable of handling on their own.

The harsher sentence Grossberg received didn't make sense to me, nor did the fervor with which prosecutors pursued the two college freshmen. I wonder if they would have handled the situation the same way if Grossberg and Peterson had not been upper middle class, white, and from good families. What I do know are the medical findings. And they leave me with little doubt that the baby was doomed before he was even born.

Chapter Two

A FALLEN BEAUTY QUEEN

Who Killed JonBenet Ramsey?

BY DECEMBER 1996, THE NATIONAL MEDIA and the public were starting to move beyond the trial of the century in which O. J. Simpson was acquitted of murdering his ex-wife Nicole and her friend Ron Goldman. The coverage of the case and its aftermath had been nonstop, and everyone needed a rest.

But the break was short lived. The morning after Christmas marked the beginning of what continues to be perhaps an even more mysterious and tragic murder case. It grabbed the nation's attention just as spectacularly as the Simpson story, but this case wasn't about a famous ex-football player. It was about a tiny beauty queen with green eyes, blond hair, and the name JonBenet Ramsey.

The murder of six-year-old JonBenet sometime during Christmas night 1996 in her Boulder, Colorado, home has been one of the most scrutinized in recent history. Yet for all the time, money, and effort spent in trying to bring her killer or killers to justice, the case remains officially unsolved. Questions about her parents' conduct, procedures during the police investigation, and the evidence itself continue to plague the case.

My review of the medical facts and other evidence early on led me to some controversial conclusions, which I continue to believe no matter how unpopular or disturbing they may be.

●•。

The first sign that something was amiss in the Ramsey's 6,800-square-foot Tudor brick mansion was a three-page note lying at the bottom of a spiral staircase. Patsy Ramsey, thirty-nine, purportedly had awakened early the morning after Christmas and was headed downstairs from her third-floor bedroom about fifteen minutes before six o'clock to make some coffee when she found the hand-printed missive.

Mr. Ramsey,

Listen carefully! We are a group of individuals that represent a small foreign faction. We respect your bussiness [*sic*] but not the country that it serves. At this time we have your daughter in our posession [*sic*]. She is safe and unharmed and if you want her to see 1997, you must follow our instructions to the letter.

You will withdraw $118,000.00 from your account. $100,000 will be in $100 bills and the remaining $18,000 in $20 bills. Make sure that you bring an adequate size attaché to the bank. When you get home you will put the money in a brown paper bag. I will call you between 8 and 10 am tomorrow to instruct you on delivery. The delivery will be exhausting so I advise you to be rested. If we monitor you getting the money early, we might call you early to arrange an earlier delivery of the money and hence a earlier pickup of your daughter.

Any deviation of my instructions will result in the immediate

44

execution of your daughter. You will also be denied her remains for proper burial. The two gentlemen watching over your daughter do not particularly like you so I advise you not to provoke them. Speaking to anyone about your situation, such as the police, F.B.I., etc., will result in your daughter being beheaded. If we catch you talking to a stray dog, she dies. If you alert bank authorities, she dies. If the money is in any way marked or tampered with, she dies. And you will be scanned for electronic devices and if any are found, she dies. You can try to deceive us but be warned that we are familiar with law enforcement countermeasures and tactics. You stand a 99% chance of killing your daughter if you try to out smart us. Follow our instructions and you stand a 100% chance of getting her back. You and your family are under constant scrutiny as well as the authorities. Don't try to grow a brain John. You are not the only fat cat around so don't think that killing will be difficult. Don't underestimate us John. Use that good southern common sense of yours. It is up to you now John!

Victory!

S.B.T.C.

Before Patsy Ramsey even finished reading the note, she reportedly raced upstairs to check her daughter's room. JonBenet wasn't there. Patsy screamed for her husband, John Ramsey. A quick inspection of their son's room found nine-year-old Burke safe inside. But JonBenet was nowhere to be found and John Ramsey told his wife to call 911. The call to the Boulder police department came in at 5:52 A.M.: "We have a kidnapping . . . Hurry, please."[1]

Officers arrived quickly and performed a cursory search of the sprawling mansion. But police weren't the only ones responding to the Ramsey house that morning. The Ramsey's pastor and four friends also showed up after the distraught couple called them. Instead of securing the home as a crime scene—this was a kidnapping, after all—authorities allowed the visitors access. It didn't take a seasoned detective to realize whatever evidence and other clues that may have been present could have easily been damaged or destroyed by people roaming around the residence.

Detectives did not find any evidence of a forced entry, although a kitchen door had what could have been pry marks. John Ramsey, fifty-three, told officers all the doors had been locked before they went to bed and remained so after the couple discovered their daughter was missing. Also, a small basement window was broken and a blue suitcase rested on the floor just underneath it. John Ramsey allegedly told a friend he broke it the summer before.

Several hours had passed with no word from the kidnappers when one of the detectives asked John Ramsey and his friend, Fleet White, to search the house thoroughly for anything that might be out of place. They started in the basement, and John Ramsey entered a rarely used and windowless room where some of the children's Christmas presents had been hidden. That was where, sometime about 1 P.M., he found his daughter's body.

JonBenet was covered mostly with a blanket, her mouth covered by duct tape. She was wearing a white shirt with an embroidered silver star on the chest and white long underwear from the hip to the ankle. Her arms were flung over her head. A white cord was wrapped tightly around her neck and was knotted to a wooden stick that allowed the garrote to be tightened. Another part of the cord loosely encircled her right wrist outside the cuff of her shirt. JonBenet's body was cool to the touch. Body stiffening, known as rigor mortis, already had begun to set in. She clearly was dead.

But John Ramsey tore off the duct tape from his daughter's mouth, then gathered up the girl and the blanket and carried her upstairs before placing her down on the living-room floor. It was perhaps an understandable action by a grief-stricken father, but one that caused immeasurable damage to the investigation. One of the cardinal rules when investigating a death scene is not to move the body. Valuable clues can be learned by the body's position, and other evidence on or around the body can be gathered. By John Ramsey's moving the little girl, who knows what kind of trace evidence, such as hairs, fibers, body fluids, or even fingerprints, was tainted or destroyed?

The next day, newspapers carried the story of a murdered beauty queen, which was when I first learned of the case. A picture accompanying the story in the *New York Times* showed her in heavy makeup with her blond hair teased and wearing a glitzy showgirl costume. Certainly not the image of a six-year-old girl I would have expected to see. Little did I know then that in a matter of weeks I would be examining even more disturbing pictures of JonBenet.

On January 6 I received a call from Ken Harrell, a reporter for the supermarket tabloid the *Globe*. He asked if I would review a case they were following "on the West Coast." He didn't mention the case, although he said they needed it done quickly. Eventually I agreed, but I declined a consulting fee that the tabloid offered. When dealing with the media, I don't accept payment for my services. The next day, a colleague of his flew to my office to hand-deliver a number of pictures.

I was stunned to realize they were of JonBenet's body. At that point, the only detail the Boulder County coroner had released about the case was the cause of death: asphyxia due to strangulation. Not much else had been publicly revealed about the circumstances of the little girl's death.

One photo showed the white cord wrapped around her neck so tightly it furrowed into her skin. Part of the cord was looped and knotted around a jagged piece of wood. Other photos showed the cord tied loosely to JonBenet's right wrist. These images suggested to me that someone had been playing a dangerous game that went too far.

I studied the pictures closely. To me, the way the cord was tied around her neck and wrist indicated JonBenet had been bound with the intent to restrain, not kill. The stick was connected to the cord in a such a way that it could be used as a handle with which to turn and tighten the rope. The cord around the wrist easily could have been used to keep JonBenet from resisting.

In previous autopsies, I had seen binding of a similar sort, and it was related to sexual activity. Bondage is not an uncommon fetish and can be viewed as a sexual turn-on for either those bound or those doing the binding. The use of restraints around the neck serve to decrease the flow of oxygen to the brain, creating the medical condition known as hypoxia. Men have used such bondage on themselves while masturbating, in effect slowing the oxygen flow to their brain to heighten their sexual experience.

Unfortunately, men sometimes can get carried away with the process and actually choke themselves to death in what is called autoerotic asphyxiation. As many as one thousand people a year die experimenting in this way, according to FBI estimates. In Jon-Benet's case, it looked to me as though someone had used the garrote around her neck in a kind of vicarious form of autoerotic asphyxiation. Whoever did this to her did it for his or her own sexual gratification. And given that conclusion, it wasn't a big step to believe the torture of JonBenet went hand in hand with masturbation by her assailant and/or the sexual molestation of JonBenet.

The idea that such an "adult" form of sexual role playing was used on a kindergartner made me think of the picture that accompanied the first story I saw about JonBenet's death. In it, she looked like she was six going on twenty-three. Did someone get some sort of perverted sexual thrill out of dressing JonBenet in such an inappropriate manner? After all, the somewhat suggestive costumes she wore while competing in various beauty pageants were nothing I could imagine any normal six-year-old girl would wear by choice.

I then turned my attention to the question of why JonBenet died, and if her attacker had intended solely to torture her with the use of the cord. A theory that made sense was that the rope around her neck pinched the vagus nerve, a key controller of many of the body's organs. The nerve runs from the brain down both sides of the neck and into the torso. Among other functions, it regulates the heart and lungs. If signals from the vagus nerve are interrupted, cardiac and respiratory responses could slow down, become irregular, and eventually cease—a process known as "electrical death." In normal function, special cells in the heart transmit neurological messages very quickly—reminiscent of an electrical impulse—that make the heart beat in a rhythmic fashion. If something interrupts those messages, a chain of events begins that can lead to death.

The short-circuiting of the vagus nerve doesn't manifest itself in any obvious way, so JonBenet's death would have been inexplicable to her assailant. Following through with my analysis, if the person who controlled the noose didn't mean for JonBenet to die, then the case might not be a murder as it was almost universally viewed. Her death might well have been not from an intentional strangulation, but rather the unintentional consequence of a one-sided sex game gone awry. Still a horrendous crime, but different.

An article in the *Globe* with my explanation appeared January 21, along with some of the pictures. Not surprisingly, it caused quite a controversy. Nearly everyone condemned the tabloid and expressed disgust that it would publish such graphic photos of JonBenet. There were boycotts, and a spokesman hired by the Ramseys called it "ghoulish." I did not escape the fury, either. Police and prosecutors criticized me, suggesting people in my position should refrain from commenting on the case so as to not compromise the investigation. That suggestion was nonsense. I didn't reveal any confidential material or secrets of the investigation. The comments I made were certainly not news to the killer or even details JonBenet's assailant would have expected police not to notice. However, I had no formal connection to the case and therefore had no ethical or professional duty to remain silent.

I understood the inclination of police to withhold specific details of their investigation. That can be prudent at times. But I also believed my providing information to the public was beneficial. JonBenet's death had touched many people throughout the country. Moreover, the public had a right to know about investigations into crimes such as hers.

The coroner, Dr. John Meyer, called for an inquiry into how photos from his files had been obtained. The trail eventually led to a private detective hired by the *Globe* and a technician at a commercial lab that developed the coroner's film.[2] Prosecutors charged the two, and they pleaded guilty to obstructing government operations, a misdemeanor. A judge sentenced them to three days in jail and community service, and imposed fines.[3] He also ordered the men to write a letter of apology to the Ramseys.

By then, John and Patsy Ramsey had not formally spoken with detectives. The couple had answered some preliminary questions from the first officers at the house when it appeared that there was a kidnapping. But other issues had arisen, and investigators hoped to get more answers from the multimillionaire business executive and the former Miss West Virginia. That would not happen right away. Within a week of JonBenet's death, John Ramsey hired prominent criminal defense attorney Bryan Morgan. He was a partner in the powerful and politically connected Denver law firm of Haddon, Morgan & Freeman. One of the other partners, Hal Haddon, managed former senator Gary Hart's 1974 and 1980 election campaigns and was a top adviser when Hart ran for president in 1988. Patsy Ramsey, too, retained counsel, Patrick Burke, who worked in the same law firm as Morgan. All contact by police with the Ramseys now had to funnel through their attorneys.

But the couple was not totally silent. On the first day of the new year, they appeared in the Atlanta studios of CNN for an exclusive interview. The family was in Georgia, where they lived when Jon-Benet was born and where they had returned to bury her.

They told reporter Brian Koebel that both of them had given blood, hair, and handwriting samples to authorities, as well as fingerprints.

"There is a killer on the loose," Patsy Ramsey said, on the verge of tears. "I don't know who it is. I don't know if it's a he or a she.

"But if I were a resident of Boulder, I would tell my friends to keep . . ." She began crying and after a moment continued, ". . . to keep your babies close to you. There's someone out there."

At one point, the interviewer asked the Ramseys about speculation on talk shows casting suspicions on them. "It's got to be sickening," he said.

"Oh, it's nauseating beyond belief," John Ramsey said.

"You know," his wife added, "America has just been hurt so deeply with the tragic things that have happened. The young woman [Susan Smith] who drove her children into the water. And we don't want what happened with O. J. Simpson. I mean America is suffering because they have lost faith in the American family. We are a Christian, God-fearing family. We love our children. We would do anything for our children."

The two said they decided to speak out to thank the countless people who had helped them and prayed for them during the past week. The couple also wanted to plead for help in solving their daughter's death and announced that they were offering a $50,000 reward for information leading to JonBenet's killer.

Koebel questioned John and Patsy Ramsey about why they had hired attorneys. "Most laymen who don't understand would say, 'Why? You're grieving parents. You want to find somebody? Why an attorney?'"

"Well," John Ramsey said, "it's not just an attorney. We are also assembling an investigative team to assist. I want the best minds this country has to offer to help us resolve this. This doesn't come from anger. It comes from knowing that the only way my family can move on now is to resolve who and why this happened."

He added that the Boulder police had been wonderful and were working hard. The couple recounted the morning of December 26, from Patsy Ramsey's finding the ransom note to John Ramsey finding JonBenet's body. She said she answered questions from police all that day, and when Koebel asked if they would be willing to sit down with detectives again, John Ramsey said, "Absolutely."

"We want them to know everything possible."

"Everything," his wife said. "Whatever they want. Whatever anyone wants. We will cooperate."

It would be months before that happened.

After the broadcast, Boulder mayor Leslie Durgin took issue with Patsy Ramsey's comment about a killer on the loose. She implied that there didn't seem to be evidence supporting that and the remark could do nothing but create an unnecessary anxiousness in residents. After conferring with the police chief, the mayor made her comments to the ever-growing throng of media in her town.

"There *is* a killer," Durgin said. "But I think the implication, which is completely erroneous, is that there is a murderer walking up and down the streets looking for young children. That's overlooking some pertinent facts. There was no forced entry into the home. The person who did it apparently knew the house. That does not imply to me a random act."[4]

* • •

As the case entered its second week, several elements of the investigation leaked out to reporters. One dealt with the ransom note. Detectives learned it came from an 8½-by-11-inch legal pad in the

Ramsey house. Furthermore, as was later revealed, investigators found a practice note on the page just before the three that had been torn out. Someone wrote on it, "Mr. and Mrs. Ramsey." The revelations struck me as peculiar. What kind of kidnapper would break into a family's home intent on snatching their little girl and forget to bring a ransom note? Would an assailant actually spend the time to look for something to write on and something to write with, then compose a lengthy note, all the while risking discovery? Finally, would a kidnapper forget to take the most crucial element for such a crime—JonBenet? It was almost preposterous.

The other information that trickled out from authorities was of more use to me in trying to determine what happened. Reports indicated JonBenet had suffered a fractured skull and also had been sexually assaulted. News of her molestation didn't surprise me. In fact, I would have been shocked if it came out that she had not been assaulted sexually. Based on the photos provided to me by the *Globe*, I believed molestation was the primary motive behind the whole incident. It was one of my first thoughts after seeing the rope around her neck with the attached piece of wood and the binding of her wrist. Binding is often connected with sexual activity, and the stick in the tourniquet was a way to control someone. An assailant wouldn't need something that elaborate if all he wanted to do was strangle a child.

The skull fracture, however, was a twist that I didn't anticipate. If the purpose of the assault on JonBenet was sexual in nature, I wasn't sure how a violent blow to her head became part of the scenario. How could the girl who was chosen Little Miss Colorado months before her death provoke such an action? I was hoping more information might offer some clues. And the one document that could reveal the most details was the autopsy report.

Unfortunately, a judge had sealed the report in early February based on assertions by the coroner and district attorney's office that disclosing such specific information could damage the investigation. It contained details that only the killer would know, they argued. But Colorado law provided that an autopsy report be open to the public unless authorities could show "extraordinary circumstances" justifying its sealing. A legal battle ensued when lawyers for the media became involved and a middle ground was reached: on February 14 a judge ordered the partial release of the report—seven pages with some redactions. The remainder of the document would remain sealed for another ninety days or after an arrest, whichever came first, the judge concluded.

I received a copy of the edited report from the *Globe* and eagerly read through it. On the last page under the heading "vaginal mucosa," I found the facts to back up my initial theory about what happened in one succinct paragraph: "All of the sections contain vascular congestion and focal interstitial chronic inflammation. The smallest piece of tissue, from the 7:00 position of the vaginal wall/hymen, contain epithelial erosion with underlying capillary congestion. A small number of red blood cells is present on the eroded surface, as is birefringent foreign material. Acute inflammatory infiltrate is not seen." Essentially, someone had used an object to penetrate JonBenet's vagina and in doing so left behind telltale signs of abuse.

During his microscopic examination of thin tissue samples taken from internal membranes of the vagina, the coroner, Dr. Meyer, found vascular congestion and focal interstitial chronic inflammation. Vascular congestion is merely more blood than normal in certain vessels, which was a natural response to the pressure or injury that had caused the inflammation. Focal interstitial meant there was inflammation in some spots in the walls of the vagina, but "chronic" was the key word that caught my attention.

In the world of forensic pathology, chronic means at least forty-eight to seventy-two hours old. There's no fudging that time frame, which meant the injury didn't happen around the time of Jon-Benet's death. It didn't even happen hours before she died. The damage was inflicted *days* before. Had Dr. Meyer found indications of a more recent injury, he would have described it as "acute," but that wasn't the word he used.

Dr. Meyer's discussion of the piece of tissue from the lower left portion of the vaginal wall (the seven o'clock position) described how the chronic inflammation had caused part of the lining to deteriorate and erode. The inflammation also caused the capillaries underneath that area to become congested with blood.

This seemed to me to be at least a partial explanation for the coroner's reference under his final diagnosis, which included an "abrasion and vascular congestion of the vaginal mucosa." Further description of the abrasion he described apparently had been edited out in the initial version of the autopsy report released to the public.

Dr. Meyer further noted a small number of red blood cells on the eroded surface. The area must have suffered an injury or trauma that forced those cells out of their normal home, the blood vessels. It was a sign of an acute injury, something that had happened shortly before JonBenet died. So there were signs not only of chronic abuse, but also of more immediate, acute trauma in the same area.

The coroner also observed in that area of the vaginal wall birefringent foreign material, which becomes visible under the microscope when exposed to polarized light and observed through a blue prism. It commonly contains silica, which is a component of lubricants such as talcum powder. The possibilities for how something like that got into JonBenet's vagina ranged from sinister—perhaps a lubricated rubber glove worn by a molester—to benign—talcum powder used to soothe an irritated genital area.

Taken as a whole with the acute and chronic injuries, however, it seemed fairly clear something had been inserted into her vagina over a period of several days. A finger seemed the most likely intruder, based on the evidence. A digit inserted from someone's right hand and then curled to rub against the vaginal wall would make contact at just about the seven o'clock position.

Dr. Meyer's final comments in the section were that he found no acute inflammatory infiltrate. That would be white blood cells, the body's soldiers that rush to the scene of an injury. Usually it takes an hour once damage occurs for those white blood cells to arrive. The fact that Dr. Meyer found none told me JonBenet died before they could get there.

Overall, the injuries documented in the autopsy report all pointed to sexual abuse. Nothing I reviewed suggested this could have been the result of a natural condition such as a bladder infection or chronic bedwetting. Considering all options, I couldn't rule out masturbation, but I felt it was highly unlikely. It just didn't seem logical that a six-year-old girl would be masturbating at any point, much less in the moments before someone tightened a garrote around her neck and cracked her skull.

Many months later I learned Dr. Meyer had reached essentially the same conclusion. In an affidavit from one of the police detectives that was included in court documents, the investigator wrote that Dr. Meyer told her JonBenet "had received an injury consistent with digital penetration of her vagina."[5]

The redacted autopsy report also included some details about JonBenet's head injury and other marks on her body, as well as Dr. Meyer's examination of the internal structure of the girl's neck. The coroner found a scalp contusion that was associated with the fracture. Upon removing the skull, he noted a subdural hemorrhage and a subarachnoid hemorrhage, which were collections of blood underneath the dura membrane, a thicker, tougher layer closer to the skull, and the arachnoid membrane, named because of its spider web–like pattern. Obviously, the blow to her head had caused the internal bleeding.

Dr. Meyer further referenced another brain injury: small contusions on the tips of the temporal lobes. The temporal lobes are located behind the temples on the side of the head; bruising of them can occur from being shaken. The brain literally slides slightly inside the skull and bangs up against the bone, creating bruises. I believed that that was more likely than some external injury in that area of the head because the report didn't describe any such overlying external trauma.

In fact, the shaking fit quite logically with my theory that JonBenet's assailant didn't intend for her to die. Once the sex game involving the tightening of the ligature around her neck went beyond the point of no return, I had no trouble believing whoever controlled the noose shook JonBenet in a desperate attempt to get her to regain consciousness.

I found more support of an unintentional death in the coroner's dissection of JonBenet's neck. A thorough examination of all layers of the neck is especially important in strangulation cases. In this case, the strap muscles—those that run along the sides of the neck—showed no sign of hemorrhage. That was one sign the choking was not intentional.

Other clues were found deeper in the neck. The U-shaped hyoid bone at the top of the throat was not damaged. Neither was the thyroid cartilage, which is the Adam's apple, nor the cricoid cartilage, which is the uppermost ring of the trachea. These structures often are damaged during strangulation, especially from manual asphyxiation. The absence of trauma indicated to me that the garrote around JonBenet's neck was, in theory, supposed to be carefully controlled.

There were more minor abrasions found on the rest of JonBenet's body. One, about three-eighths of an inch long and one-quarter inch wide, was behind and just below her right ear. Others were on her right cheek, the back of her right shoulder, two on her lower left back, and one on the lower back of her left leg. They all were consistent with JonBenet squirming on the unfinished concrete floor, if on her back, or the rough concrete walls, if she was standing against one of them. This squirming likely would have occurred during the sexual abuse and tightening of the ligature.

Dr. Meyer's review of the internal organs did not reveal much more, but I was interested to learn that she had only a small amount—about two teaspoons—of unidentified thick mucous material in her stomach. In the upper part of her small intestine, however, there were bits of what the coroner believed to be pineapple. It takes about two hours for food to move from the stomach to the small intestines, so finding out when JonBenet ate the pineapple could help narrow the time of death.

As it was, determining a time of death was difficult in this case, made even harder by the fact that the coroner didn't view JonBenet's body at the scene until 8:20 P.M., nearly seven hours after she was found. The sooner a forensic pathologist can inspect a body for crucial details such as rigor mortis (body stiffening), livor mortis (blood pooling), and algor mortis (body cooling), the better the chance he or she can narrow the time of death.

In response to written questions submitted by police, the Ramseys and their attorneys wrote back that JonBenet "may have eaten some seafood, such as cracked crab and/or shrimp" at a friend's party Christmas night. The pineapple must have been eaten once the family returned home, but their answer didn't mention pineapple. Interestingly, investigators found a bowl containing the fruit on a breakfast table in their house. It had Patsy Ramsey's fingerprints on it.[6] She later denied feeding JonBenet anything that night after they got home.

After the partial autopsy report was released, JonBenet's pediatrician spoke out, rejecting the idea that she had been sexually abused. Appearing on *PrimeTime Live*, on September 10, 1997, Dr.

Francesco Beuf said that in the past three years JonBenet had complained of pain while urinating in three of her twenty-seven visits. The girl's vaginal inflammation was due to poor bathroom hygiene or irritation from bubble bath, the doctor believed. Dr. Beuf said he probably would have found the vaginal injuries discovered during the autopsy if they had been there during his exam, but he wasn't certain. That's because he didn't perform a full gynecological checkup, which is rarely needed and performed on a six-year-old.

●　•　●

As each turn of the police investigation into JonBenet's death was reported in the press, a side issue in the case also had taken on a life of its own. It was the beauty pageants that JonBenet had participated in, the source of many of the images splashed in newspapers, magazines, and television. In one shot she's in sequins, high heels, and more makeup than a Las Vegas showgirl. In another, she stares at the camera with her blond hair tousled, looking like a Charlie's Angel.

I had no doubt that JonBenet's participation in these contests may have played a role in what happened to her. Dressing a six-year-old girl in scanty outfits, coating her with makeup, and then sending her on stage to prance around was offensive and inappropriate. The transformation of JonBenet into a pseudoadult set up an unhealthy sexual undertone in regard to this child.

I realize that there are supporters of these pageants. They argue that the contests are not only fun for the girls, but also help them with issues of self-esteem and shyness. Moreover, the youngsters make new friends with other contestants, and pageants provide girls and their mothers with something they can do together. Those are all admirable qualities, but there are plenty of other activities—sports or other types of talent shows—that provide the same benefits without putting the little girls on display in such a questionable manner.

59

Many agree with me. One of the most prominent is Marilyn Van Derbur Atler, Miss America 1958. Van Derbur Atler, who disclosed that she had been the victim of incest by her father, served as a consultant to Boulder police and prosecutors within months of JonBenet's death. She always opposed little miss pageants, knowing the girls were learning that they would be rewarded if they were beautiful, if they had perfect bodies, and if they could appease the desires of other people.

"What the JonBenet cycle of beauty pageants does, in my opinion, is set them up for major cosmetic surgery, eating disorders, an obsession about how they look, why they're loved, who likes them—those kinds of things," Van Derbur Atler said. "And it's the wrong message, in huge block print."[7]

● • ●

As the investigation continued, the Boulder County district attorney's office became more involved. D.A. Alex Hunter held a news conference February 13, 1997, relaying his hopes of solving the case and how he had assembled what he called an expert prosecution task force. It soon became known as the prosecution "dream team," a play on the group of attorneys and experts who worked for the defense on the O. J. Simpson case. Ironically, the team included two members of O. J.'s defense crew, defense attorney Barry Scheck and forensic scientist Dr. Henry Lee.

Before concluding, Hunter made some comments directed specifically at JonBenet's killer. "The list of suspects narrows. Soon there will be no one on the list but you," the prosecutor said, referring to the unnamed murderer. "You have stripped us of any mercy that we might have had in the beginning of this investigation," he continued a short time later. "We will see that justice is served in this case, and that you pay for what you did. And have no doubt that that will happen."

I watched the press conference on TV in a hotel suite in Pittsburgh. With me was a crew from *Inside Edition*, a program for which I had agreed to act as a commentator. There was a minor problem, though. Hunter hadn't really said anything new. I was glad to hear he had my distinguished friends Barry Scheck and Dr. Henry Lee on the case, but lots of questions remained. To me, perhaps the most noteworthy of Hunter's comments was his phrase about the killer having "stripped us of any mercy that we might have had." It seemed odd that prosecutors and police investigators would ever have had mercy for anyone who invaded a family's home and slaughtered a young child. Or for a pedophile who molested a little girl and then snuffed out her life.

But what about someone who knew the girl and was close to her, perhaps even her parents? Would Hunter have mercy for someone like that?

Almost as soon as Hunter announced his office was stepping in with both feet, the district attorney's office and Boulder police were at odds. In the ensuing months and years of the investigation, prosecutors would bemoan purported mistakes by police detectives and claim the investigators didn't listen to them. Conversely, police would accuse prosecutors of sabotaging their efforts and inappropriately sharing critical evidence with the Ramseys' team of attorneys. More than a few observers have argued that the inability of prosecutors and police to work together on the case contributed mightily to its failures.[8]

Part of Hunter's plan involved bringing in Lou Smit, a retired homicide detective who had worked for the Colorado Springs police as well as the El Paso County sheriff's office and that county's district attorney's office. Smit was well respected by law enforcement officials, and I doubt Hunter had any idea where the veteran cop would eventually stake his allegiance.

Smit initially set about immersing himself in the volumes of reports, witness interviews, and evidence that investigators had collected and which were now being kept in what was supposed to be a secure "war room," or headquarters for the probe. One interesting piece of information was that while authorities were able to rule out John Ramsey and others as the author of the ransom note, they could not do the same for his wife. They examined a handful of samples she submitted, as well as other writings, deemed to be unrehearsed, that police had seized from the Ramseys' summer home in Michigan. Experts hired by the Ramseys and their attorneys, however, contended that there were too many discrepancies between Patsy's writing and that on the note.

Additionally, investigators concluded that the black felt-tip pen used to write the ransom note came from inside the house.[9] And the amount of the ransom demand—$118,000—was the exact amount of John Ramsey's bonus that year, a fact known to only a few people.

As winter turned to spring, detectives still had not been able to schedule a formal interview with the Ramseys. The two sides could not agree on ground rules; both blamed each other for the problems. Separate interviews had been set for John and Patsy with Smit, Hunter, and others (but not with anyone from the Boulder police). Authorities as a group would have two hours with each of the parents and there would be a two-hour break during which both could talk with their attorneys.

Police Chief Tom Koby called off the sessions, a day before they were supposed to occur, on the advice of the FBI, which considered the conditions for the interviews set by the Ramseys to be unacceptable and damaging to the case. The Ramseys' attorneys responded with a letter to the district attorney. It accused Boulder police of conducting a "cowardly smear campaign against John and Patsy, fueled by leaks and smears attributable only to 'sources.' We will no longer endure these tactics in silence."[10]

The interviews eventually took place, but before they did, the

Ramsey attorneys got copies of police reports, the ransom note, and photo negatives of certain evidence. Their attorneys also were able to examine the garrote used on JonBenet.[11] In the end, Patsy Ramsey spoke with detectives for a total of six and a half hours on April 30; John Ramsey followed and was questioned for more than two hours.

The next day, the Ramseys held a highly controlled news conference with seven hand-picked reporters in a special room at the Boulder Marriott hotel. The journalists in the room were given conditions: they were not allowed to ask about the specific details surrounding JonBenet's death or the police interviews of John and Patsy Ramsey. Both parents denied killing their daughter.

"To those of you who may want to ask, let me address very directly: I did not kill my daughter JonBenet," John Ramsey said. "There also have been innuendos that she has been or was sexually molested. I can tell you those were the most hurtful innuendos to us as a family. They are totally false."

When I later heard John Ramsey's comments, I had to shake my head. From the portions of the autopsy report that already had been released, I believed there was no question someone had molested JonBenet. This wasn't a forcible rape with penile penetration, but something—a finger or other object—had been inserted into her vagina. Of that, I had no doubt. And in mid-July, I became even more convinced.

That was when additional sections of the coroner's autopsy report were released. It contained more details about Dr. Meyer's vaginal examination. The latest disclosure revealed that he found a small amount of dried blood along the edges of the labia major, the outer lips of her vagina, and near the skin area between the vagina and rectum called the perineum. More dried and semifluid blood also was found on the tissue between the outer and inner lips, known as the fourchette, as well as in the entrance to the vagina, called the vestibule.

On the inside of the vestibule, the coroner noted reddish discoloration due to hyperemia, essentially congestion of blood in the vessels of the vagina and vaginal wall. The congestion was "circumferential," an indication to me that whatever caused the mark had moved in a circular motion. A finger perhaps? That made sense. Dr. Meyer also found a faint violet discoloration on the right outer lip of the vagina, which appeared to be a superficial bruise, and a small amount of semiliquid, thin, watery red fluid inside the vaginal vault.

In the earlier release of autopsy information, the coroner documented a one centimeter red-purple area of abrasion in the seven o'clock position at the opening of the hymen. Now a previously redacted portion showed a significant portion of her hymen was gone. A rim of tissue between the two o'clock position and the ten o'clock position was what remained.

One doesn't have to be a forensic pathologist to know that the hymen in a six-year-old girl should not be missing, even partially. Some sports or other strenuous activities can damage the hymen, but JonBenet was not a horseback rider and had not been riding a bicycle shortly before her death. This was winter in Colorado, after all. I also had to consider the other evidence here: fresh blood in the vagina, abrasions, a chronic inflammation, and some sort of foreign material in the vagina. Those conditions are not found in little girls who are running around a playground.

As revealing as the new disclosures were about the injuries to JonBenet's vagina, the latest section of the report provided even more details about the skull fracture she had suffered. It was a blow so massive it split the bone on her head from front to back. The fracture was eight and a half inches long and went from behind her right ear, up and forward toward the top and front of the skull. Parts of the fracture were comminuted, which means some of the bone was pulverized and displaced—a clear indication of the force of the impact.

Dr. Meyer further found a roughly rectangular displaced piece of bone behind the right ear. It measured one and three-quarter inches by a half inch. That was the point of impact for whatever instrument was used to strike JonBenet and is known as a pattern injury. Forensic pathologists can make inferences on what may have caused the trauma based on that information. In JonBenet's case, a rectangular bone fragment with a fracture line running off it was indicative of an object with a handle and heavy head.

A heavy flashlight or golf club already had been suggested, and I thought those were reasonable inferences given the characteristics of the injury. What's more, whatever struck JonBenet's head didn't break through the scalp. It left a bruise but did not produce a laceration, and that was another indication that the object was rounded with a smooth edge or no edge at all.

But while her scalp was not cut, there was a wide area of hemorrhaging, or bleeding, within the scalp, spread over an area of seven by four inches. That finding seemed in line with an injury of that sort. It was what Dr. Meyer found under the skull—or more accurately, what he *didn't* find—that surprised me. From the first version of the autopsy, I already knew there was a subdural hemorrhage (subdural meaning underneath the dura, a tough fibrous membrane between the brain and the skull). However, the most recent disclosures revealed the hemorrhage was a thin film of only about seven to eight cubic centimeters of blood. That's, at most, two flat teaspoons.

I would have expected substantially more subdural bleeding with an injury as significant as JonBenet's skull fracture. The minor bleeding told me that she had a weak, and possibly nonexistent, heartbeat when her assailant struck her. If the heart was barely pumping at the time, it would not have had enough pressure to deliver blood to the injured area of her head. She must have been nearly dead or in the agonal stage, the moments just prior to clinical death. Why else would there be so little blood at the site of the fracture? The amount Dr. Meyer found is what I considered residual blood, generally blood that remains in small vessels after the heart has stopped beating.

The coroner also must have considered that likelihood. He listed the cause of death as "asphyxia by strangulation associated with craniocerebral trauma," not the other way around. Additionally, the autopsy report listed the ligature strangulation injuries first, followed by JonBenet's head trauma.

But the order of her injuries made me wonder why JonBenet's attacker would crack her head open when it must have appeared that she was already dead. I went back to the idea that the entire incident was some sort of devious sexual game with unintended consequences. If the pressure on JonBenet's vagus nerve from the ligature had short-circuited her breathing and heartbeat, she would have been rendered unconscious. Staring at a limp and lifeless little beauty queen, JonBenet's molester may have panicked and decided to create, outwardly at least, an obvious reason for her death. He or she may have thought that the rope around her neck was not enough to attribute the death scene to some intruder. Something with more brutality was needed. Thus the massive skull fracture.

I also considered the possibility that the injuries happened in reverse—she was hit on the head first and then the garrote cinched around her neck, yet the theory didn't work from a medical standpoint. Had the head injury occurred initially, there would have been much more hemorrhaging, or bleeding, in the layers between the brain and the skull. While JonBenet undoubtedly would have been knocked unconscious, she would not have died immediately. The area of the brain that controls her heart and lungs would have continued to function, sending a steady supply of blood to her head.

Another point to be considered in determining which injury came first was brain swelling. Dr. Meyer's observations during the autopsy regarding the size of JonBenet's brain was used as an argument against my conclusion that she was at death's door when struck in the head. I couldn't agree with the reasoning. The coroner weighed her brain and found it had swollen to 1,450 grams. That is about 15 percent heavier than the 1,200 to 1,250 grams that one would normally expect in a child such as JonBenet. The swelling must have come from the blow to the head, the argument went, meaning she would have had to live longer than I suggested was probable.

But a brain that is deprived of oxygen also swells. If the game of vicarious autoerotic asphyxiation was being played out and the noose tightened, the amount of oxygen getting to JonBenet's brain would be decreased. The brain would have reacted within seconds to the hypoxia, or lack of oxygen, and have begun swelling.

Finally, to dispel the reverse-order idea on a more common-sense level, why would anyone use a garrote and rope around her wrist—after the fact—as a way to confuse investigators? I felt it was much too elaborate a scenario. Still, there were other physicians whose conclusions differed significantly from mine.

I found that out in the days following the release of the autopsy report's second portion on July 14, 1997. The two major newspapers in Denver, the *Rocky Mountain News* and the *Denver Post*, had been covering the story extensively. Both included comments from Dr. Richard Krugman in their stories on the latest autopsy report information. Dr. Krugman, a pediatrician, was dean of the University of Colorado School of Medicine and had been advising District Attorney Alex Hunter on the case. He also was a nationally recognized expert on child abuse and did not believe JonBenet had been sexually abused.

"I know nothing that I have seen that would make me think the primary finding is sexual abuse," Dr. Krugman said in the *News*. "I look at this and see a child who was physically abused and is dead. I don't believe it's possible to tell whether any child is sexually abused based on physical findings alone."

He viewed the injuries to JonBenet's vagina as "mild trauma." The injuries, he said, could have been indications of irritation from bubble bath or an infection, and were not sufficient to make a diagnosis of sexual abuse. That type of abuse usually can be corroborated by the presence of semen, evidence of a sexually transmitted disease, or a review of the child's medical history.

Dr. Krugman told the *Post* he couldn't tell whether JonBenet's death was due to strangulation or her head injury. But the skull fracture did tell him that she had suffered from "an explosion of rage."[12]

The *Post* also quoted Dr. Todd Gray, the chief medical examiner for Utah. Dr. Gray said he believed JonBenet had been strangled after the blow to her head, and the petechial hemorrhages (the pinpoint hemorrhaging of very small veins), among other evidence, proved she was alive at the time the garrote was tightened around her neck. "This wasn't a gentle killing; this kid was fighting," he told the newspaper.[13]

I found their interpretations hard to square with the evidence in the autopsy report: blood inside and around the vagina. There shouldn't have been any blood. A good portion of the hymen of a six-year-old girl was missing. Signs of chronic and acute inflammation in the vaginal wall. Some sort of foreign material in the vagina. The indications of sexual abuse and some sort of vaginal penetration were abundant and apparent to me.

I also could not agree with Dr. Gray's conclusion that JonBenet was strangled after suffering the skull fracture. It is quite clear the head injury was so massive that it would have caused unconsciousness, if not death. So how could she have been fighting after that?

But not everyone held a contrary opinion. Further articles included comments from Dr. Ronald Wright, who at the time was director of forensic pathology at the University of Miami School of Medicine. Dr. Wright, who also had served as medical examiner in

Broward County, Florida, told the *News* there were obvious signs JonBenet had been sexually abused.[14] The "birefringent foreign material" found in her vagina—a substance that commonly contains silica, a component of lubricants such as talcum powder—was consistent with penetration by someone wearing rubber gloves, he said. When taken with additional information that had surfaced— that JonBenet's body had been wiped down by her assailant—the two findings argued against a typical child molester. Dr. Wright, however, sided with Dr. Gray on the order of injuries: skull fracture, then strangulation.

☀ ● ☀

The final portion of the coroner's autopsy report was released August 13, 1997. It contained descriptions of the clothes JonBenet was wearing: white long underwear that were urine stained; panties with printed rose buds and the word "Wednesday" on the elastic band, which also were urine stained; and the shirt with the embroidered silver star. But it wasn't the urine stains that caught my eye. JonBenet had been known to wet her bed, so she may have urinated involuntarily or as a way to rebel against her molester. The urine also may have been expelled after her death when the body's muscles go slack.

What got my attention were several red areas of staining that the coroner found on the inner part of the crotch of her panties. I assumed that the stains were blood, a logical conclusion given the blood found on the outside of her vagina. (I later learned Dr. Meyer had told a police detective that the stains appeared to be consistent with blood.) But what kind of sexual abuser undressed a girl, molested her, and then redressed her? That didn't fit the pattern of the many random sexual assaults I had seen. Why would an intruding pedophile who also had slaughtered a six-year-old girl care about whether her panties were pulled back up? Someone who had a connection with the girl, on the other hand, someone who cared about her, may have wanted to save some dignity for the now dead JonBenet.

The report further described the wooden stick that was used to twist the garrote. It was four and a half inches long and looked as if it had been broken on both ends. The tan stick also had several colors of paint on its surface, along with the word "Korea" printed in gold letters on one end. The details were interesting, but the real significance of the stick wasn't clear to me until some time later, when the *Denver Post* reported that it was part of a long-handled artist's paintbrush taken from Patsy Ramsey's painting supplies in the basement of the house.[15] The other sections of the handle were found in the art kit, according to the paper.

While that didn't mean much on its own, it made me consider other items involved in the attack and the supposed kidnapping plot that had been linked to the Ramsey house. In addition to the paint-brush section, investigators determined that the notepad and pen used to write the ransom note came from inside the house. Whoever committed this crime seemed to be extremely lucky to have stumbled upon all the tools necessary to carry out the plan. Or maybe the assailant knew about these things because it was an inside job.

The fact that John and Patsy Ramsey were considered suspects in the death of their daughter was established fairly soon in the investigation. The words eventually used by authorities were that they remained "under an umbrella of suspicion." But as the months passed, they and their team of attorneys and investigators suggested alternatives that deflected the spotlight away from the Ramseys.

Former FBI profiler John Douglas was one of the experts brought into the case by the Ramseys. He talked with John and Patsy Ramsey, their attorneys, and the police, and came away asserting they were not involved in JonBenet's death. Instead, Douglas suggested that officials look for the girl's killer in the circle of individuals around John Ramsey's business, such as a disgruntled former employee.

The profile composed by Douglas suggested that the killer may have been someone who had been in the Ramseys' house previously.[16] The assailant most likely was a man who might have been under stress in the weeks prior to the attack. The actual crime may have been committed to vent his anger, perhaps even at a female close to him. Following JonBenet's death, her assailant may have intently watched or read news of the crime, might have increased his consumption of alcohol or drugs, and might have tried to appear cooperative with investigators if they interviewed him.

But another retired FBI profiler, Gregg McCrary, did not agree with Douglas's interpretation of the case. Many of the elements raised in the profile could apply to any murder, McCrary believed. It didn't account for what McCrary saw as the obviously staged crime scene and the fake ransom note.[17] Still another eminent former FBI profiler, Robert Ressler, questioned Douglas's work on the case and agreed with McCrary that the ransom note was staged to cover up the identity and motive of the real killer. That killer, Ressler told the *Denver Post*, probably was someone from JonBenet's immediate circle, such as a relative, friend, neighbor, or worker in the house.[18]

Dr. Henry Lee, whom the district attorney's office had consulted on the case, also suggested to investigators that they look for suspects within the family or someone close to the Ramseys. After being apprised of the evidence detectives had gathered and the findings of the coroner, Dr. Lee brought up the idea I had believed was the most likely scenario—that JonBenet's death was accidental and some staging or cover-up had followed.[19]

That didn't deter the Ramseys, however. They had run newspaper ads in the past offering $100,000 for information that would help solve JonBenet's killing. Now, in the summer of 1997, they ran another ad with information from Douglas's profile and distributed bright orange fliers in the neighborhood. Another ad focused on the ransom note and displayed several of the distinctive letters found in it, asking people who recognized the writing to contact the Ramsey tip line.

But the efforts didn't seem to generate the response that the Ramseys had hoped for. One of their defense attorneys, Hal Haddon, told the *Denver Post*, "As far as public reaction to the ads, it's been a disaster. All the feedback from the public has been pretty negative. Everything we've said has been turned against us."[20]

* * *

While I felt the available evidence that had been made public strongly indicated an inside job, prosecutors in the case actively pursued other theories. The Ramseys passed along plenty of names of people they considered potential suspects—friends, neighbors, and former coworkers of John Ramsey's at Access Graphics. Detectives questioned them, asked for handwriting samples, and in some cases requested blood and hair samples. The leads went nowhere.

A glimpse into the thinking inside the investigation, at least from the district attorney's office, came in May 1997 in the form of a motion filed by Deputy District Attorney Bill Nagel. The motion had to do with an attempt by prosecutors to keep certain search warrants under court seal. Nagel wrote that "nothing has been discovered which would unequivocally eliminate them [John and Patsy Ramsey] from suspicion, and they remain a focus of the investigation. However, there remains the real possibility that the murder was committed by an intruder, and that possibility continues to be a serious and ongoing focus of the investigation as well."

A big supporter of the intruder theory was Lou Smit, the retired detective who had been brought in as a special investigator for the district attorney's office. Initially, Smit saw JonBenet's parents as probable suspects. But his view changed over time, and Smit eventually came to believe a different scenario, one that involved a deadly intruder. Smit resigned from the case in September 1998, convinced the Ramseys were innocent, but he continued working with the evidence that he believed showed something else.

His theory essentially was this: JonBenet's killer slipped into the house through a basement window on Christmas night while the Ramseys—John, Patsy, JonBenet, and Burke—were at a friend's holiday party. Alone, the intruder had time to familiarize himself with the large and labyrinthine mansion, find a notepad and pen to write out a ransom note, and then lay in wait. Once the Ramseys returned, the killer waited until they all had gone to sleep, then snatched Jon-Benet from her bed, using a stun gun to subdue the little girl. The attacker brought JonBenet to the basement where the assault and murder occurred, even though the predator had planned to take her from the house. The garrote and sexual assault were part of an autoerotic fantasy. When JonBenet awakened and screamed, her attacker bludgeoned the girl, then fled out the same basement window.[21]

Smit's explanation contained several points I found to be unlikely, although I thought it was interesting he adopted some of the concepts I had been talking about for years. While our ultimate conclusions differed, I noted Smit also believed the garrote tightening around JonBenet's neck and the sexual assault were connected to some sort of autoerotic asphyxiation by proxy. He also agreed with me that the skull fracture came second, based on the small amount of blood in her head, an indication that she was near death when struck.

But I felt other components of Smit's theory were much less persuasive, and in the case of the stun gun idea, medically improbable. Police had pursued the possibility that a stun gun was used in the crime, but it never amounted to anything. Investigators also consulted with Dr. Michael Dobersen, the coroner of Arapahoe County in Colorado, who had done previous work examining stun gun injuries. At the time, Dr. Dobersen told detectives that the abrasions on JonBenet could have been from a stun gun or they might have just been scratches. However, years later, after looking at more evidence from Smit, Dr. Dobersen became more convinced the abrasions were from a stun gun.

The impetus behind the push, and Smit's belief, were autopsy photos taken of injuries on JonBenet's body. The coroner described one mark just below the girl's right ear on her cheek as a small "rust colored abrasion," and two more on her lower left back as "dried rust colored to slightly purple abrasions."[22]

Smit said the two marks on her back and their distance from each other matched the prongs of a particular brand of electric stun gun, the Air Taser. He also felt size and shape were consistent with marks left by such an instrument, which is used by pressing its dual prongs against an individual and activating an electrical charge. But when I looked at the pictures, I didn't see that at all. For one thing, the sizes were different, and that alone should have refuted the stun gun contention. The coroner described one as three-sixteenths of an inch by one-eighth of an inch and the other as one-eighth by one-sixteenth of an inch. The coloration of the marks also varied, leading to the conclusion they weren't left in a simultaneous fashion by one object. The differences were even clearer on the marks by her face. Another point I remembered from the autopsy report was that JonBenet was wearing a long-sleeved shirt, yet no defects were found on her clothing that corresponded with the abrasion found on her back underneath it.

Other forensic pathologists also believed the stun gun theory was questionable. Dr. Werner Spitz came forward in March 2000, soon after Smit went public with his interpretation of how the crime occurred. During a previous interview with ABC News, John

Ramsey said no expert had contradicted Smit's conclusion about a stun gun. When Dr. Spitz heard that, he decided to speak out on *Good Morning America* about the abrasions.

"First of all, they were described in the autopsy report as abrasions," Dr. Spitz told Jack Ford, the show's cohost, on March 21. "They look like abrasions from what I saw. They do not look like any sort of burn. They simply don't look like an electrical burn. The one on the jaw had a pattern within it, which suggests that this is an imprint of something like a snap, you know, a snap like a button. These things just don't look like Taser marks, anyway no Taser marks that I've ever seen."

He disagreed with my conclusions regarding the sequence of injuries to JonBenet, but I nonetheless was glad to see another experienced forensic pathologist challenge the scenario set forth by Smit and the Ramseys. And don't forget that Dr. Meyer, the forensic pathologist and the one who personally observed the injuries, described them as abrasions. He made no mention of a stun gun or burns, or even hinted at the possibility in his autopsy report.

The rest of Smit's intruder theory also was wanting, in my view. To accept it, one would have to believe that a homicidal pedophile broke in through a basement window carrying a satchel of dastardly devices—a rope to use as a garrote, a stun gun, and some duct tape to silence JonBenet. But somehow he forgot a stick to tighten the ligature with, as well as a pen and pad with which to write a ransom note. How comfortable would an intruder have felt traipsing around inside the Ramseys' house looking for these items when the homeowners might have returned at any moment or already were home?

In my experience, hardened sexual predators don't leave phony ransom notes when their intent is to molest and murder. Likewise, kidnappers don't generally sexually assault and kill their targets, then leave the bodies behind. Their targets are worth more alive than dead. And what about the many ridiculous aspects of the

75

ransom note? Who asks for just $118,000—an amount that happens to be the same as John Ramsey's bonus—from a multimillionaire? And what kind of "small foreign faction" uses words like "attaché" and "hence" in a rambling ransom note?

I further questioned the suggestion that the basement window was used as an entrance and exit point, with a suitcase beneath it acting as a step. It was a small window, and an intruder would have had to squirm his way inside. I thought it likely that such a person would leave some trace of himself behind—clothing fibers in the window casing, a footprint on the suitcase, something. But none of those items were recovered.

Investigators, however, did find some other intriguing bits of evidence. In the room where JonBenet's body was discovered, there also was a shoe print from a Hi-Tec boot. Neither John nor Patsy Ramsey owned footwear that matched, but that brand is popular with law enforcement officials, and there were plenty of officers in that area during the investigation. In a book by the Ramseys, published in November 2000, they argued the boot print was one of many pieces of evidence that suggested an intruder was their daughter's killer.[23]

One of the others was a palm print found on the door that led into the room containing JonBenet's body. It wasn't from the Ramseys, and for a long time, the person who left it remained unidentified. As it turns out, there were explanations for both the palm print and the shoe print. Investigators were able to match the palm print on the door to Melinda Ramsey, JonBenet's older stepsister (from John Ramsey's prior marriage). She was in Georgia the night of the murder and cleared from suspicion very early in the case by the police. As for the print found on the floor, the *Rocky Mountain News* printed a story in August 2002 quoting police sources as saying it came from Burke Ramsey, JonBenet's brother, who was nine years old at the time of her death.[24] Authorities had also cleared the boy of any involvement in his sister's death and said the print was left prior to the incident.

Although the Ramseys' latest attorney, Lin Wood, did not dispute the palm print, he dismissed any suggestion that the boot print came from the younger Ramsey. "Burke Ramsey does not and has never owned a pair of quote, unquote, trademarked Hi-Tec sneakers that the Ramseys are aware of," Wood told the *News*. "I would think they know what shoes he has owned."

At the time, Wood pointed out other findings that still could not be explained: unidentified male DNA found in JonBenet's panties, and the ransom note. I had talked with Dr. Henry Lee many times over the years regarding the DNA issues in the case. Both of us felt it likely there was some sort of contaminant throwing off the results. In other words, the DNA could have gotten there in any number of ways that had nothing to do with her sexual assault and killing. Several years passed before a likely scenario regarding the DNA was disclosed by anonymous investigators in a November 2002 article in the *Rocky Mountain News*. Instead of the genetic material having been deposited during some sort of attack on JonBenet, it could have just as easily been left when her panties were manufactured.[25]

Authorities working on the case secured what the newspaper called "unopened control samples" of the same underwear produced at the same factory in Southeast Asia. Tests then were conducted on the samples, and some had human DNA in them. It was an illuminating analysis, but not entirely shocking to me. Human DNA—saliva, skin flakes, hair, and even sweat—can be transferred in the most innocent of ways. As the *News* suggested, even a worker's cough at the underwear plant could be enough to cause some sort of DNA contamination.

In the Ramseys' book, John Ramsey mentioned the unidentified DNA found in his daughter's panties and wrote that he believed the genetic material came from her killer. When the *News* asked the Ramseys' attorney about the anonymous authorities' latest theory, Wood called it "pretty spectacularly imaginative."

While the DNA issue seemed to me to be mired in questions about its origin and the reliability of the samples, there was other forensic evidence I felt was more compelling. Tiny fibers.

Investigators located the red fibers in Patsy Ramsey's paint tray in the basement. It was from the same tray where the broken paint-brush used in the garrote was taken. Detectives also recovered similar fibers tied into the ligature around JonBenet's neck; on the blanket she was wrapped in; and most curiously, on the sticky side of the duct tape used to cover her mouth. Authorities believed the fibers came from a red and black jacket Patsy Ramsey was wearing the morning of JonBenet's death.[26] She also was seen wearing the same piece of clothing in pictures taken at the Christmas party the night before.

Prosecutors asked her about the fibers during questioning in August 2000, a follow-up to previous interviews John and Patsy Ramsey submitted to with authorities. The Ramseys eventually provided videotapes of those sessions to the CBS program *48 Hours*, which broadcast a program about the case October 4, 2002.

"I have no evidence from any scientist to suggest that those fibers are from any source other than your red jacket," special prosecutor Bruce Levin told Patsy Ramsey during the videotaped interview.

An answer came not from Ramsey, but from her attorney. "Well, again, that's—come on. I mean, they—what other sources did they test?" lawyer Lin Wood asked. Wood wanted prosecutors to show him the evidence, but they would not, and the attorney didn't let Patsy Ramsey respond to Levin.

But two years later, when she appeared before the cameras for *48 Hours*, Patsy Ramsey had an answer.

"After John discovering [*sic*] the body and she was brought to the living room, when I laid eyes on her, I knelt down and hugged her. But I was—I had my whole body on her body. My sweater fibers, or whatever I had on that morning, are going to transfer to her clothing," she told the program's correspondent, Erin Moriarty.

On first blush the answer sounded logical, even probable. Clearly with someone who was that close to JonBenet, a transfer of clothing fibers would be expected. So if the blanket that was placed over JonBenet after she was brought upstairs was the one the prosecutor referred to, I understand that the finding does not seem relevant. But if the assistant district attorney was referring to the "death blanket"—the one from JonBenet's bed that she was wrapped in when found in the basement—then that's a different story. John Ramsey acknowledged leaving that white blanket downstairs in the room where JonBenet was found dead.

The same held true for the black piece of duct tape. John Ramsey's first act upon discovering his daughter was to rip the tape off her lips. He left that in the basement, too. So my question is this: how did red fibers purportedly consistent with Patsy Ramsey's jacket get on the sticky side of duct tape found on her dead daughter's mouth, in a paint tray, and potentially on a blanket, when Patsy Ramsey was never in the basement that morning?[27] Another question I have about Patsy Ramsey's comment on *48 Hours* relates to the garrote. Why, if all she did was hug her dead daughter, were those red fibers *tied into* the ligature? Fibers are inanimate objects. They don't act like worms and burrow into things.

A year before the *48 Hours* interview, in the spring of 2001, Lou Smit tried to provide a further explanation of evidence already in the record when he appeared on NBC's *Today* show on May 1. Host Katie Couric asked him how a neighbor of the Ramsey's could hear a child's cry between midnight and 2 A.M. from the Ramsey house the night of the murder, yet the scream went unnoticed by JonBenet's parents. Smit said the girl had been taken to a boiler room in the basement that was within ten feet of a vent pipe, which led outside the house. He claimed the pipe acted as a megaphone and funneled the sound toward the neighbor's house. In experiments with others, Smit said people at the neighbor's home could hear noises from that area of the basement while the sounds could barely be heard by people in John and Patsy's bedroom on the third floor.

When I heard this, I was reminded of one of my favorite quotations. It is from Sherlock Holmes and, I thought, quite appropriate. "Once you eliminate the impossible, whatever remains—no matter how improbable—must be the truth."

It wasn't just the scream that John and Patsy Ramsey didn't hear. It wasn't just the ransom note with its foreign faction and other nonsensical phrases. It wasn't just the problems associated with squaring the evidence with an intruder. And it wasn't just the inconsistencies of John and Patsy Ramsey's statements with the facts in the case. No, it was all those things and more that led me to consider the comment of England's most famous fictional detective.

After eliminating the improbable, I was left with two adults in the house that night—JonBenet's parents. I cannot say with certainty the exact scenario that led to JonBenet's death on that cold winter night in the bowels of her home. But I believe the evidence could support charges against both John and Patsy Ramsey. That appears unlikely, however.

A grand jury was impaneled to hear evidence in the case in September 1998. The jurors listened to testimony and other evidence in secrecy for more than a year. The grand jurors heard evidence from police, Burke Ramsey, John Ramsey's two grown children from a previous marriage, and others. JonBenet's parents were never called. Then late in the afternoon of October 13, 1999, District Attorney Alex Hunter made an announcement at a press conference. "The Boulder grand jury has completed its work and will not return. No charges have been filed," he said. "The grand jurors have done their work extraordinarily well, bringing to bear all of their legal powers, life experiences, and shrewdness. Yet I must report to you that I and my prosecution task force believe we do not have sufficient evidence to warrant the filing of charges against anyone who has been investigated at this time."

After that, the investigation wallowed. But three years later, in December 2002, Hunter's successor as district attorney, Mary Keenan, began an in-depth review of the case. She wrote a letter December 20 to the Ramseys' attorney, Lin Wood. In the letter, Keenan strongly implied the new investigation would not focus on the Ramseys as suspects.[28] But it also said the latest inquiry would not exempt them.

Chapter Three

SEX, DRUGS, AND A DEAD CASINO MAGNATE

How Ted Binion Died

L AS VEGAS HAS LONG HELD A reputation as a place of excess and extremes. It is a place where mobster Bugsy Siegel built a resort called the Flamingo Hotel, and later, where the Rat Pack set up camp.

In Sin City, anything can happen. And quite often it does.

That held true in the case of casino magnate Lonnie Ted Binion, whose family owned the Horseshoe Club casino and whose partially clothed body was found on the floor of his sprawling home the afternoon of September 17, 1998. What followed was a bizarre story that touched on buried millions, nineteenth-century Scottish killers, organized crime, infidelity, drugs, and charges of murder.

Perhaps this is par for the course in Las Vegas. But it turned out to be one of the more intriguing cases I have investigated in the past decade. It also was one in which I believe the outcome was not supported by the medical evidence.

After studying the case—the autopsy, the pictures, police reports, tissue samples, Binion's prior statements, and the statements of others—and testifying in the trial, I am convinced that the authorities had it wrong. Unfortunately, some rather routine tests and other actions that could have helped provide clearer answers about Binion's death were never performed.

It all started with a brief, frantic phone call to 911 shortly after 4 P.M. on September 17, 1998. "My husband's not breathing," a woman said, and then the line went dead. The dispatcher was able to trace the call, and when paramedics arrived at Binion's ranch house, they found a hysterical Sandra Murphy waiting for them outside. She quickly led them to the southeast den.

Binion, the flamboyant casino executive, was lying face up on a sleeping mat, his hands at his sides and his legs straight out. A comforter was partially draped over his lower body. He was dressed only in underwear and a striped dress shirt that was pushed up on his chest. An empty prescription bottle for the antianxiety drug Xanax was on the carpet nearby, as were three disposable lighters, an opened pack of Vantage cigarettes, and a remote control for a television or VCR. It didn't take emergency workers long to determine that Binion, fifty-five, was dead.

But beyond that, the scene did not immediately hint at what might have happened. Police officers and crime scene analysts, who descended on the house within an hour, saw no obvious signs of foul play. Binion did not appear to have been shot or stabbed, and the area around his body was not ransacked or disturbed, as one might expect if there had been a violent struggle.

The most that investigators observed at the scene were a few slight abrasions on Binion's body. One was on the back of his right hand and another on the front of his left knee. A reddish mark in about the center of Binion's chest also was noted.

A search of a nearby bathroom, however, revealed some clues.

On a small stand next to the toilet, authorities found a pocketknife with a brownish residue on the blade, an ashtray, and a clean piece of foil. In the trash can were several pieces of crumpled foil and a piece of pink rubber balloon. Another scrap of balloon, this one red, was found on the floor. Those are signs of drug use. Another indication that Binion's death may have been drug related was the empty bottle of Xanax found next to his body. It was dated September 16, a day earlier, and was for 120 0.5-milligram pills. Two weeks would pass before results of toxicology tests came back showing lethal levels of heroin and Xanax in Binion's system.

As police investigated inside Binion's house, friends who had heard about what happened and others interested in the goings on lingered outside. The gathering of such a crowd wasn't surprising, given Binion's colorful life and the reputation he had built. He was a man who carried huge wads of cash with him—usually about $4,000, but on occasions, many tens of thousands of dollars—and also, almost always had a gun strapped to his body. He slept with a shotgun near his bed, hid $250,000 in a boat engine in his house, and was friends with reputed mobsters.

I came to learn more about Binion and his history after Sandra Murphy's attorney asked me to consult with him on the case and review the evidence in early 2000. By then, Murphy, twenty-seven, and the man authorities said was her lover, Rick Tabish, thirty-five, were facing murder charges, accused of orchestrating Binion's fatal overdose.

Ted Binion, as he was known, was one of five children. His father, Benny Binion, was a cowboy from Texas who ran bootleg liquor and some gambling operations before moving his family to Las Vegas.[1] Once in Sin City, the elder Binion opened the Horseshoe in the early 1950s, and the casino quickly became known for setting higher limits on bets than other local gambling establishments.

While I have been to Las Vegas many times, I've visited the still-operating Horseshoe only once, and that was back in 1960 when I was twenty-nine. At the time I was in the Air Force at Maxwell Air Force Base in Montgomery, Alabama, home of that military branch's war college and a large hospital. On weekends I used to hitch rides with pilots who needed to keep up their flying hours and managed to visit places from Panama to Puerto Rico to all over the United States. That's how I made my first visit to Las Vegas, and it was then I walked into the Horseshoe. The casino isn't on the Strip, where many of the more famous hotels such as the Dunes or the Sands are located, but rather is in the downtown section of Las Vegas. Since I'm not a big gambler, I didn't place any bets.

The Horseshoe was a family operation, and Ted Binion earnestly followed his father, mother, and older brother into the business when he was twenty-one. He dealt blackjack and counted the slot drop. A year later, in 1965, he acquired an ownership interest in the Horseshoe. The younger Binion seemed to have a knack for gaming, and he soon became the casino manager.

Ted and his brother Jack, who was casino president, brought the World Series of Poker to the Horseshoe in 1970. In the early years, anyone could enter, and that drew amateurs and professionals alike, including gambling legends such as Amarillo Slim Preston and Johnny Moss.[2]

But Ted Binion's skill in managing the casino eventually was overshadowed by a major problem—his addiction to heroin.[3] Binion first tried the drug when he was nineteen and used it occasionally to get high during the next couple of decades. Mostly, according to his former wife, he smoked marijuana. By the early 1980s, however, as even Binion later acknowledged, he had become a heroin addict.[4] He wasn't able to function effectively as casino manager and in time stopped working. He spent his days at the house heating heroin on tinfoil and then inhaling the smoke, a process known as "chasing the dragon."

Binion's addiction continued for years until the problem came to a head in 1987, when police arrested him on heroin trafficking charges. The case was resolved after he pleaded guilty to lesser charges and was placed on probation. But the criminal case caused repercussions in Binion's professional life. The Nevada Gaming Commission also put Binion on a probation of sorts, effectively suspending his gaming license for six years.

For parts of the next decade, Binion was subject to periodic drug testing and failed at various times. His gaming license was suspended again in 1997 because of his admitted drug use, and finally revoked by the state's Casino Gaming Control Board in March 1998. At the time, control board officials cited Binion's drug charges from a decade earlier and his connections with alleged mob figures. One of them, Herbert Blitzstein, who was alleged to be involved with a crime organization out of Chicago, was killed in January 1997 over what authorities believed was a Mafia turf war. Additionally, Binion admitted loaning $100,000 to another man with supposed mob ties.[5]

Given that Binion's drug use and his battles over his gaming license were highly publicized in the Las Vegas newspapers, detectives who responded to his house the evening of September 17, 1998, must have been aware, at least in passing, of that history. When they spoke with Binion's live-in girlfriend after his death, they learned more. Sandra Murphy, who met Binion in 1995 while she was working as a dancer at a topless club, told them Binion had been trying to kick his heroin habit and was considering entering a drug treatment facility. She also said that he had been depressed about his drug use and threatened suicide, putting the barrel of a handgun in his mouth several times while high.

Later on the night of Binion's death, police talked with reporters about the situation and they publicly knocked down any suggestions that Binion had been murdered. "Preliminary results indicate he may have made an ingestion error in regards [*sic*] to medication," Las Vegas police Sgt. Jim Young told the *Las Vegas Review-Journal* for a story that ran on the front page the next day. He went on to say, "At first glance, it appears accidental and not an intentional act. While it's suspicious, it's not suspicious to the point where we are talking about criminal activity."[6]

Young gave essentially the same comments to the *Review-Journal*'s rival, the *Las Vegas Sun*, which also quoted homicide Lt. Wayne Petersen as saying, "There was absolutely no evidence at the scene to suggest foul play."[7]

Petersen no doubt was responding to one of Binion's sisters, Becky Behnen, who told the *Sun* that night she felt the case "should be treated as a homicide until proven otherwise."[8]

The next morning, Dr. Lary Simms, the chief medical examiner of Clark County, performed an autopsy on Binion. He noted many of the same marks on Binion that had been observed when the body was found:

- two 2-inch-by-1-inch curvilinear contusions, or bruises, on the back,
- an irregular erosion 0.4 inches in diameter in the middle of the chest without evidence of antemortem hemorrhage—bleeding prior to death—and a smaller similar mark slightly higher on the chest,
- small patterned abrasions on the right wrist of parallel superficial lines 0.4 inches long, and
- some discoloration on the right side of his nose and in the area just under his nose and above his upper lip.

Dr. Simms dissected Binion's neck organs but found no perihyoid, perilaryngeal, or peritracheal hemorrhages—bleeding within certain areas of the neck that he most likely would have seen had Binion been strangled. The medical examiner also checked

Binion's lower eyelids and the conjunctivae (the membrane lining the inner eyelids) for signs of petechiae, or pinpoint hemorrhages—often another indication of strangulation. While there was vascular congestion, or a bit more blood in the blood vessels there, he found no petechial hemorrhages.

About a week later, Dr. Simms studied some tissue samples he had taken from a bruise on Binion's back, which showed hemorrhaging without a vital reaction. In essence, that indicated that the bleeding had occurred a short time before or even after death. But perhaps the most telling part of the autopsy were the toxicology tests. The results showed what police initially suspected—Ted Binion died of a drug overdose. Testing indicated he had in his system morphine, which is a breakdown product of heroin, alprazolam (Xanax), and diazepam (Valium).

That tied in with what police detectives had learned. The Xanax prescription came from Dr. Enriq Lacayo, a physician who also was Binion's next-door neighbor. The doctor told police he had treated Binion in the past and prescribed the Xanax at Binion's request. Binion told Dr. Lacayo he was anxious and had been trying to stop drinking and taking drugs. Binion believed that the Xanax would help him get off heroin.

Detectives also spoke with a man who said he delivered twelve balloons of black tar heroin to Binion the night of September 16—less than twenty-four hours before Binion was found dead—in exchange for $240 and about thirty Xanax pills. It was the largest amount of heroin Binion had ever purchased from the man.

On Binion's death certificate, dated October 2, 1998, Dr. Simms listed the cause of death as alprazolam and opiate intoxication. The manner of death, however, was listed as "pending police investigation." That's exactly what they were doing. By then, detectives were taking a closer look at Sandra Murphy and her relationship with Binion. So was a private investigator hired by Binion's family.

Authorities also were interested in Rick Tabish, who had befriended Binion earlier in the year. During the summer of 1998, Tabish was one of several people who helped Binion move about $7 million of Binion's silver bars and coins from the Horseshoe to the garage of Binion's home. Binion eventually hired Tabish to build an underground cement vault on Binion's ranch property in Pahrump, about forty-five miles west of Las Vegas.

Two days after Binion was found dead, a sheriff's sergeant patrolling Binion's ranch at about 2 A.M. came across Tabish and two other men. One of them was operating an excavator. Inside a tractor trailer at the ranch was about twenty tons of Binion's silver. Tabish explained he was removing the silver so he could sell it and give the proceeds to Binion's daughter. But officials were skeptical of the story and arrested him and the two other men on charges of burglary and grand larceny.

●　•　▪

Another nine months passed before police arrested Sandy Murphy and Rick Tabish on charges of murder, conspiracy, and robbery. In a lengthy affidavit, detectives laid out their investigation. The document cited interviews, phone records, and medical evidence in support of the theory that Murphy and Tabish killed Binion to get some of his vast fortune. Coins, silver, and currency were missing from Binion's home after his death.

Three months before the June 24, 1999, arrests, the coroner held a press conference to announce he had changed the manner of death in Binion's case to homicide. Clark County coroner Ron Flud, Dr. Lary Simms's boss, was not shy about revealing that he believed Binion was killed. But he would not discuss what prompted him to change his decision or how authorities suspected Binion may have been murdered.

90

However, it was likely that at least part of the reason for the change had to do with the findings offered by Dr. Ellen Clark, a forensic pathologist from Reno, Nevada. The coroner's office asked Dr. Clark to review the autopsy report, photos of Binion, and other materials in the case. Dr. Clark agreed that Binion died of a multiple drug overdose and concluded the disproportionately high levels of morphine and Xanax in his stomach indicated oral ingestion of both drugs. That squared with later-revealed conjecture by authorities that Binion was somehow forced to take the lethal doses of drugs as opposed to smoking the heroin.

She also noted the abrasions above Binion's upper lip were consistent with his face having been vigorously rubbed or cleaned prior to paramedics arriving. The fact that Binion had no vomit on him was another indication that suggested to her that his body had been cleaned.

Additionally, Dr. Clark believed the livor mortis, or blood pooling, and pressure patterns on Binion's face suggested that his body was face down for a period of time after death and later moved to the face-up position. Her alternate theory was those changes in Binion's face could have occurred prior to death, if he had been subject to trauma in the form of sustained pressure.

Finally, the injuries on Binion's knee, chest, and wrist appeared to Dr. Clark to have happened *after* Binion's death—another indication his body may have been moved before emergency personnel got to the house.

"Based upon observations that the body and death scene were tampered with, that the drugs which killed Mr. Binion were ingested in an atypical fashion, and that inconsistent accounts of events preceding and immediately following Mr. Binion's death have been reported by the individual who discovered the body [Murphy], it is my opinion that another person or persons were involved in the death of Lonnie Binion," Clark wrote.

Throughout the police investigation, the private investigator hired by Binion's family also worked on the case. In fact, detectives used many of the interviews conducted by private investigator Thomas Dillard and other evidence he gathered as part of their case. Dillard also contacted Dr. Michael Baden, director of the New York State Police Forensic Sciences Unit, who had spent twenty-five years working in the New York City medical examiner's office. Dr. Baden, who I mentioned is also a close friend of mine, agreed with the local coroner that Binion's death was due to "homicidal poisoning." But Dr. Baden reserved his final opinion until he had a chance to examine the scene, autopsy photos, toxicology records, and other physical evidence.

That opportunity came August 18, 1999, when Dr. Baden flew into Las Vegas to testify at a preliminary hearing in the case. In Nevada, a justice of the peace presides over such hearings in criminal cases to determine whether enough evidence exists for them to be forwarded to district court for further proceedings. One day earlier, the preliminary hearing began against Murphy and Tabish, as well as four others accused in the attempted theft of the buried silver and a separate extortion plot.

Court officials anticipated a crush by the media, but the turnout was less than expected. One cable channel aired the entire preliminary hearing and only local papers staffed the hearing each day with reporters. The *Las Vegas Review-Journal* noted a writer from *Playboy* was in town doing research, but authorities knew the actual trial was where the most media attention was likely to be focused.

On the first two days of the preliminary hearing, prosecutors called witnesses who testified about the relationship between Murphy and Tabish—which the district attorney wanted to show was a romantic one—and Murphy's expectation that she would receive millions if Binion died. Binion's will stipulated that Murphy would receive $300,000 in cash and the house they shared, worth about $900,000.

While that was going on, Dr. Baden visited the medical examiner's office and looked over tissue slides and viewed more photos. He also was taken to Binion's house by Dillard, the private investigator, to examine where Binion's body was found. When he finally sat down in the witness box the afternoon of August 19, what Dr. Baden had to say stunned both defense attorneys and courtroom observers.

"The cause of death was asphyxia by suffocation. That is inability to breathe by, because of suffocation," Dr. Baden said in response to a question by the prosecutor.

"Taking into account that opinion," Deputy District Attorney David Wall then said, "the marks that you described on Mr. Binion's chest, the discoloration or marks that you observed around his mouth area, the marks that you observed or the trauma that you observed on both the left and right wrist, observation that you made and photographs that you've seen regarding the scene of the crime, and the bruises not only to the back but the hemorrhage in the front lower chest area, are you able to take all of those into a scenario which accounts for each of those facts as it relates to the cause of death?"

"Yes," Dr. Baden replied.

"And what would your opinion be?"

"My opinion would be that the marks on the wrists would indicate some kind of restraint at some point prior to death," Dr. Baden said. "That the findings about the mouth and chest are typical for [a] type of suffocation that's called Burking."

Reading a transcript of Dr. Baden's testimony some months later while preparing my findings on the case, I was rather surprised to see that he was relying on a rarely used diagnosis that dates back to the 1820s in Edinburgh, Scotland. The manner of suffocation was named after a man, William Burke, who along with a collaborator, William Hare, spent time digging up bodies from graves to sell for anatomical dissection.[9] To cut down on their work, the two decided to pursue living victims.

They started by getting their mark drunk. Then Burke would sit on the person's chest, an act that prevented the lungs from expanding and caused mechanical asphyxia. At the same time, Burke would cover the victim's nose and mouth to suffocate him. For the purposes of Burke and Hare, this method was seen as most efficient because it left no obvious marks on the victim. But his method wasn't foolproof, and Burke eventually was hanged for his deeds.

Dr. Baden further testified he believed this was how Binion died and based his opinion partly on the abrasions on Binion's chest. He said they were consistent with imprints that would have developed from shirt buttons if there was a downward pressure on them. Dr. Baden also believed those abrasions would have occurred within half an hour prior to Binion's death. The contusions (bruises) on Binion's back probably happened within the same time frame, Dr. Baden said, and could have come from a hard surface such as a floor or from a fist. He found further proof for his theory in Binion's lower eyelids, where he said he found petechial hemorrhages, or pinpoint ruptures of blood vessels that can occur in suffocations.

I was even more surprised to learn of Dr. Baden's other conclusions in the case. He said the drug levels in Binion's system were not lethal. In fact, Dr. Baden didn't even think Binion would have passed out from the amount of heroin and Xanax he had ingested. (He said that he came to his earlier conclusion after reviewing a report that had a typographical error regarding the amount of Xanax in Binion.) "I think as far as the drug overdose, which was Dr. Simms's opinion, in my experience the amount of drugs that Mr. Binion had in his system could cause death, but the great majority of people who have that amount would not die from the drugs," Dr. Baden said during the preliminary hearing. "It was very low levels."

After listening to two weeks of testimony, Justice of the Peace Jennifer Togliatti ruled there was enough evidence for the case to move forward. At the same time, she made a point of mentioning there was not a great burden of proof required in a preliminary hearing.[10]

● ● ●

In January 2000 attorney John Momot contacted me. Momot represented Murphy and wanted me to review the case. I agreed, and by the end of February I was on a plane to Las Vegas to meet with them, to examine preserved tissue samples at the coroner's office and to tour Binion's house to see where he died.

They also asked me to answer some three dozen questions about Binion's death, the marks on his body, and the drugs in his system. A couple of the most pertinent queries pertained to whether Binion was suffocated, as Dr. Baden testified, or died some other way, and the effectiveness of investigators' methods in determining Binion's approximate time of death.

Murphy's defense team was struck, as was I, that prosecutors were pursuing two seemingly mutually exclusive theories—either Binion was forced to overdose or he was drugged and then suffocated. I always thought of the legal unacceptability of such a courtroom presentation as what law school students and professors refer to as "Horn book" law, or traditionally accepted law. This was not a game where the butler stabbed him in the kitchen or the maid shot him in the bedroom. It's one or the other, and allowing a jury to consider both theories in the Binion case seemed to me confusing and unfair.

I arrived in Las Vegas the evening of February 24 and checked in at the Golden Nugget Hotel. As I mentioned, gambling doesn't really interest me; I don't have the patience for it and I'm practical enough to realize I probably won't come out a winner. Besides, I had work to do, spending several hours the next morning at the coroner's office.

There I examined the tissue slides and found the medical examiner's descriptions of his findings to be essentially accurate. I did note that Binion's lungs together weighed 1,412 grams, a little more than three pounds. That's at least double the lung weight normally found in someone of Binion's overall weight of 157 pounds. What was causing the disparity became clear under the microscope. The tissue slides of the lungs showed vascular congestion and significant pulmonary edema.

Vascular congestion means the blood vessels in Binion's lungs were engorged with blood. The pulmonary edema goes along with that. The phrase refers to the noncellular or serum component of blood. It's a proteinaceous fluid that is forced out of the congested vessels because of pressure and into the alveoli or air sacs of the lungs. The congestion and edema are rather classic findings in a drug overdose death. But they are not things you would expect in a case of "Burking."

In the afternoon, I went to Binion's house to examine the surroundings. Even though seventeen months had passed since his body was found there, I still believed it was important to get a sense of the scene. In virtually all death investigations, a review of the scene can provide invaluable clues. Sandy Murphy met the defense team and me at the house. She was dressed simply, and I noticed she seemed rather small.

Sandy met Binion in 1995 while she was working at a topless club named Cheetah's, and within months she moved into Binion's house, after Binion's wife moved out. "I had a good feeling about her from the very first," Binion said about Murphy in 1996, during a deposition for his divorce proceedings.

Murphy described to me how she found Binion and the position of his body, as well as other details about their usual sleeping arrangements. She sometimes slept in a separate bedroom from Binion; his ex-wife noted separately that he snored loudly.

● • ●

Later I looked at pictures of Binion at the scene to determine whether his body might have been moved after death, as Drs. Simms and Clark suggested. They based their opinions on discolorations on Binion's face that they believed were an indication of lividity or blood pooling.

When a person dies, the blood in their body obviously stops circulating. If the body remains in the position it was in at the time of death, gravity begins to take effect within half an hour to two hours. That causes blood to pool in dependent parts of the body, or areas closest to the ground. Within eight to twelve hours, what is called livor mortis becomes fixed, meaning even if the position of the body were changed, the characteristic reddish purple markings would stay. The process is quicker in warmer conditions, and paramedics did find Binion with a comforter draped over part of his body.

In her report, Dr. Clark suggested the marks on Binion's face could have come from the onset of livor fixation while his body was face down, but that it later was moved to its face-up position. I saw some purplish discoloration, but on the right side of Binion's face near his ear. The mark there made perfect sense to me, considering Binion's head was tilted slightly to the right in the pictures taken at his house. However, I did not see other evidence of lividity anteriorly—on the front of Binion's body—or any other indication that his body had been moved.

Investigators at the scene rolled his body over, which revealed moderate purple-red discoloration with pale areas on his upper back, and crease marks left by his shirt. Pictures taken the next morning at the autopsy showed marked and more thorough lividity without crease marks. That told me lividity was still developing when the pictures were taken at the scene. Such a difference can help narrow the estimated time of death, but it still isn't completely accurate.

Death investigators also can look at rigor mortis, or body stiffening after death, to help establish a time frame. Parts of the body become stiff as the muscles' energy source is depleted. Typically, this begins to happen within half an hour to two hours after death, first in the smaller muscles such as the jaw, before gradually evolving throughout the body. In violent deaths, such as a soldier on the battlefield, in cases of physical exertion, or in situations in which the body is in a warm area, rigor mortis can set in much quicker.

But normally rigor mortis sets in fully within six to twelve hours after death. An investigator with the coroner's office noted at 4:40 P.M. rigor mortis had set in Binion's jaw. I believe Binion could have died as soon as three to four hours earlier, or as long as six to eight hours before. A convenience store clerk said Binion bought cigarettes at about 5 A.M. September 17, and his neighbor's maid testified that she saw Binion about forty minutes later, barefoot and looking as if he had just gotten up.

By the accounts of those witnesses, it's obvious Binion could not have died any earlier than about 6 A.M. And if one of Binion's friends is to be believed, she said she called just after noon on September 17 and spoke with Murphy, who told her Binion was out of it and couldn't talk. Murphy then went to lunch with Tabish and one of his attorneys. According to Murphy, when she returned back to the house, she found Binion unresponsive.

In the end, the closest I was able to establish a time of death, based on the medical evidence, was anywhere between 8:40 A.M. and 2:40 P.M. that day.

Those are estimates, however. Real life isn't like television or novels, where coroners are able to divine magically the exact time of death. Forensic pathologists generally have to deal with ranges of time in unattended deaths, especially in this case, because of the variations that can occur with livor mortis and rigor mortis.

There are, however, at least two more reliable methods used to narrow the time of death. Unfortunately, one was not used and the other performed too late in this case. Had they been done or performed in a more timely fashion, everyone could have had a more specific idea as to when Binion died.

One has to do with body cooling, or algor mortis, and can be helpful in situations in which a person has been dead fewer than eight hours. It involves taking the core body temperature at the scene with a special thermometer that is inserted into the liver or sometimes high into the rectum. Another reading is taken some time later, usually at the coroner's office, to get more reference points to help establish a more specific time of death. Given that bodies generally cool about a degree and a half in the first hour after death and a degree or so each subsequent hour, this method allows a death investigator to figure out the rate of cooling and fix a narrower window than with livor mortis or rigor mortis.

The other technique entails taking a reading of potassium levels found in a fluid behind a deceased person's eyes. It also has its limits, and the procedure loses its usefulness on bodies that have been dead more than twelve hours. The investigator withdraws the eye fluid, known as vitreous humor, using a very fine needle that is inserted at the back of the eye, being careful not to touch any part of the eyeball. Then, using certain formulas to determine potassium levels in the vitreous humor, he determines a more specific time of death, usually within a couple of hours. Eye fluids were drawn from Binion, but not until the next day. By then, many hours had passed, so it was beyond the point at which the procedure is considered scientifically reliable in narrowing the time of death.

The photos also helped me interpret the marks on Binion's body that authorities alleged were evidence of an assault. I started with Binion's back, where there were two vague, purple-red contusions more to his right side. The one higher on his back was somewhat rectangular, while the lower one was more linear and thin. I considered both to be petechial contusions, that is, they were not one large bruise, but rather multiple small ones. The marks were not patterned in any way and clearly didn't come from a fist, as had been suggested. The pinpoint bursting of small blood vessels more likely was caused by a fall against an irregular surface or something with an edge protruding from it. Not an unlikely scenario for someone stumbling around high on drugs.

A microscopic slide of one of the contusions, or bruises, showed a mild to moderate hemorrhage, but there was no inflammatory response. This means Binion was alive when the injury happened or else there would not have been bleeding under the skin. But the fact that there was no inflammatory response also means it happened close enough to his death that his body didn't begin the process of dealing with the damage. The contusion's color, reddish purple, indicated it was a recent injury. (If it had been orange, yellow, or green, that would have pointed to its being an older injury.) Based on those factors, I believe that the bruises occurred within one to two hours prior to death.

Then there were the thin linear scratches on the back of Binion's right wrist and a reddish superficial abrasion on the back part of his left forearm. That mark was just above his wrist with some pulling away of the skin. To the prosecution, those marks were an indication of some type of restraint, quite possibly handcuffs. However, I found no pressure marks around either wrist, an argument against restraints. If Binion's wrists had been handcuffed or tied up in some way, more broad and circumferential lesions would have been left. The small size of the abrasions further convinced me they did not come from restraints.

What I felt was more likely was that the marks on his wrists, along with the small reddish abrasion on his left knee, formed at about the same time as the bruises on Binion's back. Taken as a whole, all the marks were consistent with the result of a fall or someone staggering around and bumping into furniture or other fixed objects.

That left the two nearly circular marks on Binion's chest. The lower one, almost in line with his sternum, was darker colored, but both were parchment-like dull. Their coloring was an orangish brown to a dull yellowish orange. Coloring of injuries can be vital in determining when they occurred.

And in this case, the color of the erosions on Binion's chest and their parchment-like appearance indicated that they happened after death, or postmortem. The marks could have been made several minutes or several hours after Binion's death. The autopsy findings of Dr. Simms further supported my belief. Simms noted that the chest marks showed no signs of antemortem hemorrhaging, or hemorrhaging prior to death.

The configuration of the abrasions and their location strongly suggested they were made when the buttons of Binion's shirt were pressed onto his chest. But how? First I considered the methods Drs. Clark and Baden had suggested.

Dr. Clark theorized that the marks formed when Binion was lying face down, due to the pressure of his body weight against the ground and the buttons. To Dr. Baden, the impressions most likely occurred when Binion was being suffocated, or Burked, because the weight of someone sitting on Binion's chest would press the buttons into the skin.

But there was a problem with both these explanations, and it related to Binion's chest configuration. He had what is called *pectus excavatum* (*pectus* for chest, *excavatum* for excavated). Basically, he had a deep valley or inverted breast bone, a congenital condition. The abrasions were at the base of that depression. So if someone were sitting on Binion's chest, his or her weight would be distributed to the sides, not the center. The same holds true if Binion's body was face down. There's no way pressure against the buttons could have created those marks under either scenario.

There is, however, a simple and quite persuasive explanation. During the preliminary hearing, one of the first emergency medical technicians to arrive at Binion's house the afternoon of September 17, 1998, testified about a sternum rub administered to Binion. The procedure, which involves using a fist to press firmly down and rub on a person's sternum to stimulate a reaction, was in Binion's case administered on top of his shirt. That action easily could have left the marks found on Binion's chest.

●　•　●

As I examined the case further, I found more discrepancies in the prosecution's theories. One had to do with the lesions on Binion's face. It was hard to say exactly what caused them. But the marks were not patterned and were not characteristic of vigorous skin cleansing, an idea proposed by Dr. Clark. The lesions were nothing I had ever seen in smothering cases where the palm or fingers of a hand, or a soft pillow, is used. And the medical literature about Burking did not describe similar markings.

Besides, if someone applied enough pressure with his or her hand just below the nose, to leave a diffuse discoloration like the one found, there normally would be a corresponding injury to the undersurface of Binion's upper lip. But during the autopsy, the medical examiner found no damage there, or for that matter any injury to Binion's gum, teeth, tongue, or cheeks.

Another sign one would expect to find in a smothering, or in a Burking case, is lesions around the nose, but there were none. Finally, if Binion was not unconscious, as Dr. Baden suggested, I would have expected a lot more trauma around Binion's face (as well as his wrists) because he'd be putting up quite a fight. It is the most basic physiological, fundamental need of any animal to breathe, so if Binion was at all conscious—even if that level of consciousness was compromised by the drugs in his system—he would have battled against the suffocation attempt. Such injuries simply were not present.

Again, a simple explanation for the lesions may be the most probable. To me, the marks suggested nothing more than a bit of skin irritation that many men get from shaving. Close-up photos of Binion's face at the scene showed facial stubble as if he had not shaved in a day or two, a finding entirely consistent with the marks being a localized irritation.

From there, I moved on to photographs of the inside of Binion's lower eyelids. It was in those photos that Dr. Baden found what he believed to be petechiae hemorrhages, pinpoint hemorrhages that can be indicative of asphyxiation. Petechia are small, anywhere from two-tenths of a millimeter to up to two millimeters, and somewhat round. When blood backs up or becomes congested in the circulatory system, blood in the veins cannot return in a freeflowing manner to the heart. The smallest veins, called venules, then become so engorged that blood has to escape another way. When it does, petechial hemorrhages are formed. But it is important to note that petechiae can be produced from a whole host of conditions, ranging from tumors to noxious fumes to heart failure.

In cases of asphyxia, petechiae can be found not only in the lining of the lower eyelids, but also around the lips, the inside of the cheeks, and on the lining surfaces of the lungs and heart. In Binion's case, Dr. Baden noted them, but no one else saw them. The medical examiner did not see petechiae in Binion's eyes or anywhere else. What the Polaroids of the lower left eye showed me was a linear hemorrhage, quite different from the pinpoint spots of petechial hemorrhages. This one was about a millimeter wide and at least a quarter of an inch long.

Linear hemorrhages are a typical postmortem artifact—something that evolves at the time of death or afterward, but isn't associated with any specific disease or injury. Rather than being evidence of asphyxiation, the mark appeared to me to be a rather classical sign of *tache noire*—a French term describing the drying of the eyes after death. A photo of Binion's right eye showed another curved line of reddish discoloration, perhaps vascular congestion, but obviously not petechial hemorrhages.

Having gone through exactly the same photos and other evidence that Dr. Baden had investigated, I was a bit stumped as to how he arrived at his conclusion. I didn't think the evidence—some superficial abrasions here and there on Binion's body, a mild skin irritation on his upper lip, two marks on his chest, and linear hemorrhages on his eyes—was anywhere near sufficient to support a diagnosis of Burking.

● • ,

In my opinion, the medical evidence didn't add up to suffocation. I turned my attention to the drug levels in Binion's body, which was what Drs. Simms and Clark agreed killed him. The toxicology screening tested for certain drug levels in the blood and tissues of several areas: the heart blood, the peripheral blood, the liver, the gastric contents, and the vitreous fluid.

The heart blood, as might be assumed, comes from the heart. The peripheral blood is blood headed toward the brain and therefore, I believe, a more important reading, because it indicates the drug levels affecting the brain and other body tissues. The liver is where the drugs are metabolized or broken down. The gastric contents are what is in the stomach, which has not yet been digested, and the vitreous fluid is the liquid behind the eye, which takes longer to accumulate evidence of a specific drug than the liver or blood. Getting readings from the various locations can help in

Table 1: Level of Drugs in Binion's System

	Morphine	6-Monoacetyl-morphine	Alprazolam	Diazepam
Heart blood	75 ng/ml		270 ng/ml*	501 ng/ml*
Peripheral blood	88 ng/ml			
Liver	189 ng/g		124 ng/g	
Gastric contents	1,755 ng/ml	13,317 ng/ml	872 ng/ml	
Vitreous fluid	67 ng/ml	14 ng/ml	56 ng/ml	

*Test results did not specify the type of blood. Ng/ml is nanograms per milliliter and ng/g is nanograms per gram.

developing a timetable of ingestion and whether the drug levels are increasing or decreasing.

Table 1 shows the level of several drugs in Binion's system: alprazolam (Xanax), diazepam (Valium), morphine, and heroin breakdowns known as metabolites of morphine (6-Monoacetylmorphine).

All drugs have ranges that are considered therapeutic, that is, the doses in which they perform their intended medicinal purpose, as well as the ranges deemed lethal. For morphine, the therapeutic level is below 100 ng/ml and the lethal level is 50 to 4,000 ng/ml. The two ranges overlap somewhat because of differences in how morphine affects various people. Some cases of death have been documented with levels that in others would not be fatal. So Binion's peripheral blood level of 88 ng/ml of heroin was within the fatal range.

With Xanax, the levels are more pronounced. The therapeutic level of alprazolam is 25 to 102 ng/ml and the lethal level is 122 to 390 ng/ml. Binion had more than two times the highest therapeutic dose of Xanax in his system. Ingesting those amounts of either drug could have killed him, but combining the two was even worse. Throw in some diazepam (Valium), which was at therapeutic levels in Binion's body, and that just adds to the problem.

All three drugs affect the central nervous system and act to depress the brain. And since the brain controls the heart and the lungs, depressing the brain also depresses the cardiac and respiratory function. In essence, the morphine, the Xanax, and the Valium worked in concert with each other to create a more powerful and disastrous effect greater than they would have separately. That's why people taking sedatives are not supposed to drink alcohol.

With those drugs acting synergistically to slow his cardiac and respiratory functions, there was only one outcome—a slippery slope of respiratory depression leading to stupor, then coma, and finally death.

There were other questions I needed to tackle regarding the drugs. Baden estimated Binion had no more than about half a Xanax pill in his stomach, based on drug levels in the forty milliliters (about an ounce and a half) of gray-brown fluid found there. My calculations placed the number of pills in his stomach at about one and a half pills, not a big difference. The total number of Xanax pills Binion took, however, is much harder to estimate accurately.

But using a formula derived from the levels of Xanax found in Binion's blood, I believe he ingested another thirty-five to fifty pills on top of the ones in his stomach. A more accurate assessment could have been made if the medical examiner had just opened Binion's small intestine and obtained those contents for testing.

A man is found dead and next to him is an empty pill bottle dated the day before. A thorough autopsy on any potential drug overdose case in which there appears to be oral ingestion demands looking in the small intestine. That's because if pills were taken with just water or another liquid, they could pass through the stomach in less than an hour. Therefore, it's likely that inside Binion's intestine were either intact or partially digested pills, or sludge from fully digested pills. The information could have been used to determine the level of drugs, just as was done with the gastric contents.

I am certain the results would have shown even more Xanax pills than the thirty-five to fifty that I believe he had taken. Part of that belief is based on the distribution pattern of Xanax in Binion's various tissue and blood samples. The level of Xanax in Binion's eye fluid was 56 ng/ml, much lower compared to levels in the liver (124 ng/ml) and the blood (270 ng/ml). Since it takes longer for a drug to accumulate in the eye fluid than the other areas, the low levels indicate to me death occurred within a couple of hours after ingestion. It is logical then to look at the lower level in the liver and say all of the Xanax in Binion's system had not been metabolized and redistributed throughout his body.

The other issue regarding the drugs was determining how the heroin entered Binion's system. Dr. Clark believed the disproportionately high morphine and Xanax levels in Binion's stomach indicated oral ingestion of both drugs. While that seems almost certain for the Xanax, I believe it was more likely Binion "chased the dragon" and inhaled heroin smoke rather than eating it.

An article in a medical journal I found while researching the topic convinced me that I was right. The authors noted that when someone takes heroin orally, the drug is completely de-acetylated.[11] That means only morphine would be found in bodily fluids, not 6-monoacetylmorphine. But in Binion's case, 6-monoacetylmorphine was found in both the gastric contents and the vitreous fluid, which means he must have inhaled the drug.

Given the evidence investigators found in Binion's bathroom—bits of balloon, pieces of foil, and a knife with some sort of brownish residue on it—and Binion's historical use of heroin in that fashion, it's not hard to conclude that he inhaled the drug rather than ate it. The fact that no morphine was found in Binion's lungs doesn't preclude such a scenario, because the heroin smoke would be absorbed into the bloodstream almost immediately.

●　●　●

A week after my visit to Las Vegas, I submitted my report to Sandy Murphy's attorney, John Momot. In the seventeen-page, single-spaced document, I covered all the pertinent topics and concluded with my opinion:

> After completion of my evaluation and analysis of all the materials, it is my professional opinion, based upon a reasonable degree of medical certainty, that Mr. Lonnie T. Binion died as a result of a combined heroin and Xanax overdose. The distribution of heroin breakdown products (6-monoacetylmorphine and morphine) indicates that he ingested the Xanax orally, and most likely inhaled heroin smoke, also. The latter opinion is based on the type of drug paraphernalia found in his bathroom; that this has been reported as his usual method of using heroin; and finally, the lack of injection sites on his body.
>
> In my opinion, Mr. Binion ingested the Xanax intentionally, after first inhaling heroin smoke. Therefore, the manner of death would be suicide. This may have been an impulsive act, given his history of placing a gun in his mouth when "high," but it is more likely that he planned the suicide in advance. This is based on his recently having acquired large amounts of both heroin and Xanax, as well as his having isolated himself by sleeping in the den.
>
> There was minor trauma to the body that most likely was related to a fall after he became "high" (i.e., intoxicated by heroin smoke). In no way was there a distribution pattern such as to indicate that an assault had occurred, or that he had been restrained. There was also no indication that the body had been moved after

death. Lividity was only in the dependent areas; and due to the presence of pectus excavatum, the abrasions on the chest could not have been formed by the body being face down, as the sternum would have been raised off the floor.

Also if a person sat on his chest, the anterior aspects of both sides of the rib cage would have supported that individual, and there would not have been any pressure in this sternal "hollow" so as to form those abrasions. The lesions around Mr. Binion's mouth are hard to unequivocally define.

However, due to their very superficial nature, the lack of a pattern and the absence of trauma to the nose, they most likely represented a localized irritation. In no way do I believe that they indicated any attempt at smothering. Thus, I do not feel there is any evidence to support a diagnosis of "Burking."

The trial of Sandy Murphy and Rick Tabish began with jury selection March 27, 2000. The media frenzy that court officials had anticipated for the preliminary hearing had gathered some steam. Coverage of the case had been building in intensity in the weeks leading up to the trial. Some of the stories portrayed the trial as a sort of showdown between Michael Baden and me, which I found misleading and distasteful. While it was true we had reached different conclusions about Binion's death, I have been involved in too many cases, both criminal and civil, to believe juries listen only to the medical experts.

By then, both Tabish and Murphy were in custody. Tabish never was granted bail after his June 1999 arrest, but Murphy was freed pending trial after posting $300,000 bail. The conditions of bail required she remain under house arrest; and in October authorities rearrested her, claiming she violated those conditions. She was released again after a court hearing but was brought back to jail eleven days before the trial began, amid allegations of similar violations.

Opening statements in the trial before Judge Joseph Bonaventure began with Chief Deputy District Attorney David Roger telling jurors how Murphy and Tabish fell in love with each other and then planned Binion's murder. He described Tabish as a struggling businessman deep in debt and Murphy as someone who was in a position to benefit financially from Binion's death because of his will.

Still, Roger acknowledged it wasn't easy for Murphy to live with Binion, a drug addict, a known associate of "reputed mob figures," and a patron of strip clubs, who had lost his gaming license. "We're not about to paint a picture of a saint," Roger said. "However, he was a human being."[12]

He described the theories of Drs. Simms and Baden and suggested Murphy and Tabish suffocated Binion after they felt the forced drug ingestion wasn't working quickly enough. The evidence, Roger asserted, proved Binion "was murdered for lust, for greed. . . . [H]e was murdered by someone he trusted and her new companion."[13]

John Momot, however, painted a different picture of Sandy Murphy. He said Murphy got caught up in the glitz and glamour of Las Vegas, then got pulled into the "underbelly" of that lifestyle. She was a victim of Binion's powerful family, Momot said, because Binion's relatives didn't like her. But he pointed out it was Murphy who most often cared for Binion, cleaning him up after he vomited or defecated on himself while on drugs.

"This case is not about homicide. This case is about heroin. This case is not murder. This case is about money," Momot said. "This is in effect the Binion money machine at work. . . . They took this case from a drug overdose and turned it around and made it a homicide. That's what this family has done. That's what Mr. Dillard has done. Why did they do this? It's because Sandy is not a Binion. That's why."[14]

Prosecutors methodically presented their case, calling witnesses who testified about the relationship between Murphy and

Tabish, even though Momot had acknowledged one existed during his opening statements. Others testified about statements Murphy or Tabish had allegedly made about killing Binion or about his impending death from a drug overdose. One of Binion's attorneys, James Brown, testified that Binion called him the day before his death and said, "Take Sandy out of the will if she doesn't kill me tonight. If I'm dead, you'll know what happened."

The state also offered testimony about how Binion supposedly was in good spirits and looking forward to the future in the days and weeks before his death. It was meant to knock down my theory that Binion had committed suicide.

The trial continued for weeks, and after Drs. Simms and Baden took the stand, the defense team sent me transcripts of their testimony. Simms testified first and stood by his contention that Binion died after being forced to ingest a lethal dose of heroin and Xanax. But he also reiterated that he found no trauma to support the theory that Binion was suffocated.

Reading Dr. Baden's testimony, I noticed he acknowledged the bruises on Binion's back could have come from a bump against a table or a fall, but he continued to believe the marks also could have come from a fist.

Dr. Baden also minimized the finding of Dr. Simms at autopsy, and my opinion based on the pictures of Binion's body, about Binion having the inverted chest, or pectus excavatum. He said it was possible that Binion had a "slight depression." However, Dr. Baden still altered his testimony only slightly from what he said at the preliminary hearing. At the preliminary hearing, Dr. Baden testified someone probably was sitting on Binion's chest to restrict the movement of his ribcage—an action that not only led to Binion's suffocation but also left the marks from the buttons on his chest.

The statement didn't make sense to me, since I had pointed out in my report to the defense attorneys (which also was supplied to the prosecution) that Binion's quite obvious chest depression would have prevented lesions like that because the weight of an assailant would be distributed to the sides. In his trial testimony, Dr. Baden said a heavy weight such as a knee, which could fit in Binion's chest depression, was what caused the abrasions.

One month after the trial started, the defense began presenting its case. I flew out to Las Vegas on May 2, 2000, a day before I was scheduled to testify.

At the courthouse the next morning, I noticed security was tight. It also was hard to miss the TV cameras and reporters. They seemed to be all over the place.

I was the first witness called on the twenty-fifth day of the trial, and I spent the entire morning answering questions under direct examination. I used blown up images of Binion's eyelids to show the jury why the marks found there were linear hemorrhages and not petechial hemorrhages.

"This reddish line that you see on the undersurface of the eye is quite different, you can see, from a petechial pinpoint hemorrhage," I said. "I would estimate this to be about at least a quarter of an inch in length and just about a millimeter in width, but it has length. It's an area of postmortem discoloration. There it is right there, the line that goes across, which is the way Dr. Simms, who did the autopsy, described it."

I spent the rest of the morning talking about the marks on Binion's body, as well as how I arrived at my estimates regarding the time of death, and what the drug levels showed. I felt it was important for jurors to realize the powerful effect that the combination of heroin, Xanax, and Valium had on Binion.

"The brain controls everything. And when you have one drug depressing, then you have that deleterious effect," I told the jury in response to a question about how the drugs affected Binion. "When you have a second drug depressing, and then a third, you not only get the arithmetical sum of those three drugs or the pharmacological actions of those three drugs, you get an algebraic sum unpredictable, not uniformly measurable. It is a phenomenon which is referred to as synergism."

"You get a synergistic effect when you have two or more drugs that depress the brain, you get something more than two plus two equals four. Two plus two may equal 5, or 6.3, or 7.2, using numbers to connote the amount of depression that is occurring on the central nervous system. That is why every *Physicians' Desk Reference* and every package insert for all of these drugs tell you that you don't drink [alcohol] when you're taking tranquilizers, and you don't drink when you're taking sedatives and barbiturates."

"So," I concluded just before the lunch break, "now you take the morphine and you take the Xanax and you take the Valium, and you've got three drugs that are depressing the brain. . . . You have significant levels of two potentially lethal levels, a therapeutic level of a third, and you have a bad pharmacological milieu."

During the afternoon session, my testimony eventually turned to the many reasons why the prosecution's suffocation theory wasn't supported by the pathological findings. One was from a textbook I use, *Forensic Pathology* by Dr. Bernard Knight.[15] It's considered one of the best reference books on the subject in the world. In one section Dr. Knight delineates findings regarding traumatic asphyxia, that is, cases in which the chest is compressed.

"When compared to other conditions that may produce asphyxia, that particular kind of traumatic asphyxia has a high incidence of significant congestion and cyanosis [a characteristic bluish discoloration of the skin], because as it compresses the chest and doesn't permit the venous blood to come back into the heart, that venous blood gets engorged, gets backed up, and you get the bluish discoloration," I said. "I don't see any such cyanosis or marked congestion or any congestion really of any significance referred to or depicted in this case."

One of the last questions Momot asked me was why I did not believe Binion's death was a case of Burking.

"There are no injuries around the nose, around the mouth, inside the mouth, on the face," I said. "There is no congestion and cyanosis of the head, face, neck, and upper shoulder areas. There are no rib fractures or any significant injuries on the chest from that kind of pressure and force. There are no defensive wounds of any kind. The most primitive reflex of every living, thinking human being that is going to kick in automatically is the desire—the physiological need to breathe."

After a handful of questions from one of Tabish's attorneys, the prosecution began its cross-examination of me. Deputy District Attorney David Wall listed off about a dozen witnesses and asked if I had reviewed their testimony. I had not, and Wall challenged me on whether it was appropriate to reach a conclusion based on only certain bits of information.

"If I were the coroner, then I would unhesitatingly tell you, yes, I should and I would review other testimonies," I responded. "In my capacity in this case I responded to the materials that had been sent to me.

"However, it is not significant because I have no hesitation in saying to you that if I were to read the transcripts of all those individuals I might back off completely from suicide. That just takes me over to accident; it still doesn't change my opinion in terms of the cause of death and in terms of the mechanism of death and then the manner of death."

"What if I told you that some of those witnesses testified to a plot by Ms. Murphy and Mr. Tabish to kill Ted Binion using heroin and Xanax?" the prosecutor asked over objections from Momot. "Could that change your opinion of the manner of death in this case?"

"No, it would not," I said, "because I still have to deal with the medical facts and all of the physiological and pathological processes that we've been talking about."

Wall grilled me about the injuries on Binion's body, the issue of whether there were petechial hemorrhages in Binion's eyes, and the time of death. It was a thorough cross-examination, but the prosecutor did not cause me to waiver from my position.

●•●

The case was given to jurors for their deliberations on May 10, 2000. By then, the media coverage had established a familiarity with the issues. Court TV was providing "gavel to gavel" coverage, while other national cable programs such as CNN's *Burden of Proof* and Geraldo Rivera's show, *Rivera Live*, regularly featured the Binion case.

After listening to five weeks of testimony from more than one hundred witnesses, jurors had much to consider. During that time, on May 12, 2000, several people involved in the case, including myself, appeared on *Burden of Proof*. I had participated on the program in the past and found the cohosts, Roger Cossack and Greta Van Susteren, to be knowledgeable about the law and the cases they featured. Van Susteren was not on the program that day, but I was joined by Murphy's attorney John Momot, as well as a reporter for the *Las Vegas Sun* who was covering the trial, and a former state prosecutor.

Appearing from Pittsburgh, I talked about the various flaws in the prosecution's theories. I touched on why the marks on Binion's wrists could not have been caused by handcuffs and how the discoloration above Binion's upper lip was more a dermatological condition than an indication of smothering.

"All right, now, the prosecution's theory in this case and closing argument was that Binion was forced to take these lethal drugs, they didn't work quickly enough, and then he was suffocated," Cossack said to me. "You disagree with that theory."

"Yes. And, Roger, you see, that flies in the face of their own theory and much of Dr. Baden's testimony vis-à-vis, quote, 'chasing the dragon,' unquote. You get this Mexican black tar, you put it in aluminum foil, you light it on fire, and then you inhale the fumes. How do you force somebody to do that? I guess you could, maybe with a gun, but nobody ever had to force Ted Binion to take heroin.

"And then, the black tar—we found significant evidence of it in the stomach. This is a gooey, sticky stuff just like tar. How do you force somebody to chew and digest that unless you do it at gunpoint? Again, no evidence of that.

"So, the idea that this was in some way forced upon him was never, never established. It was just tossed out there and nobody ever showed how or demonstrated, nor in cross-examination was it ever put to me hypothetically in any kind of specificity, how this would have been accomplished."

Deliberations lasted for eight long days until jurors finally reached a verdict the evening of May 19, 2000. The courtroom and a nearby overflow room that had a live video feed were packed as the verdicts were read. Tabish was convicted of first-degree murder as well as ten other counts. Murphy also was found guilty of first-degree murder and five other counts.

I was disappointed after learning of the verdicts. As I've said, I had problems with the way prosecutors approached the case. They should not have been allowed to simultaneously pursue two theories as to the cause and mechanism of death—Michael Baden's Burking scenario and Lary Simms's forced overdose explanation—and then let jurors pick one. By using that approach, we'll never know if jurors separated the theories and decided guilt beyond a reasonable doubt based solely on one theory.

At a separate penalty phase of the trial, jurors recommended Murphy and Tabish each receive life with the possibility of parole in twenty years. The jury could have recommended life in prison without the chance of parole. Four months later, in September 2000, Judge Bonaventure held a sentencing hearing. Murphy received a minimum of twenty-two years in prison. The judge sentenced Tabish to a minimum of twenty-five years.

"As far as this court is concerned, this sentencing brings this case to its final chapter," the judge said in conclusion. "It is this court's desire that the victims and the families of the victims will also find some closure. Hopefully, they will be able to resume some semblance of normalcy as they move forward in their lives. As this case has garnered much media attention in this community and around the world, this court is cognizant of the fact that this community was very much affected by this case and its outcome. Now that the case has been resolved, it is hoped that Las Vegas will also find a sense of closure and return to more important matters that affect this great community. Justice, though due the accused, is due the accuser also. Justice has been served."

But in my opinion, it was not. I remain convinced that the medical evidence just does not add up to murder. It's clear to me that the injuries on Binion, which prosecutors ascribed to sinister conduct by Murphy and Tabish, could just as easily have been caused by the clumsiness of an addict who was high on heroin. And even the medical examiner agreed that Binion had lethal levels of morphine and Xanax in his system. You can't force the evidence to show something that isn't there.

There was, however, evidence that Binion had threatened suicide while high in the past by putting a gun in his mouth. I believe that after Binion inhaled heroin smoke around the time of his death he had thoughts of suicide. This time, he used what was available to him—Xanax and heroin. Given the large amount of drugs in both his stomach and his blood, an intentional overdose seems likely.

Looking back on the documents in the case, I was struck by an exchange Binion had with lawyers in his 1996 deposition.

"Would you say you have a strong-willed personality?" one of the attorneys asked.

"Not stronger than heroin addiction, no," Binion replied.

"Heroin is so addictive nobody can really do anything?"

"No," Binion said, "you have to do it for yourself."

ADDENDUM

Both Murphy and Tabish appealed their convictions, and in June 2002, respected attorney and Harvard law professor Alan Dershowitz argued before the Nevada Supreme Court that the two deserved a new trial. Dershowitz, who assisted in O. J. Simpson's defense and was working for Murphy in this case, hammered away at the prosecution's competing theories of death. He said the evidence was legally insufficient to support the murder convictions, given the disagreement among the state's expert witnesses and four defense experts' opinions that Binion died of a drug overdose.

At the hearing before the justices, one of the prosecutors said the state believed that Binion had been suffocated. Dershowitz then questioned why prosecutors called witnesses such as Dr. Simms to say a drug overdose killed Binion.

"This case should not have gone to the jury on two theories of how Mr. Binion died," Dershowitz said. "Why did the government offer the jury witnesses who said he died by a drug overdose when in this court they say it is their opinion he did not die by a drug overdose?"[16]

Dershowitz took issue with the same point that bothered me. Jurors could have arrived at their verdict by fragmentation, with some believing the suffocation idea and others the forced overdose theory.

Thirteen months later, on July 14, 2003, the Nevada Supreme

Court overturned the murder convictions of Murphy and Tabish by a five-to-two vote. In ordering a new trial, the justices did not find merit in Dershowitz's argument about the varied theories of Binion's death presented by the state. Instead, the majority ruled that a statement Binion supposedly made to one of his attorneys the day before his death and then repeated during the trial was grounds for reversal. Jurors should not have been allowed to hear the comment—"Take Sandy out of the will if she doesn't kill me tonight. If I'm dead you'll know what happened"—without the trial judge giving them an instruction about the statement. The judge should have told jurors they could consider the comment only for showing Binion's state of mind. "The prejudicial impact was great: the statement strongly implied Murphy killed Binion," the court wrote in its opinion. The justices also found another problem in the original trial that warranted a reversal. It was more complicated and had to do with prosecutors presenting evidence that Tabish and another man allegedly kidnapped, beat, and threatened a business partner of Tabish's two months before Binion died. While the state supreme court did not overturn Tabish's convictions related to those charges, the justices said there should have been a separate trial as requested by defense attorneys. To lump those allegations together with claims Murphy and Tabish killed Binion was unfair, the state's highest court ruled. As of this book's publishing deadline, a new trial had not yet occurred.

Chapter Four

THE REAL FUGITIVE

Sam Sheppard and His Wife's Murder

THE PICTURE IS IN BLACK AND white, and scrawled at the bottom is the date: June 1949. In it, a shirtless young boy is flanked by a man and a woman, who have squatted to be at the boy's level. They all gaze toward the camera, each with their own version of a smile. The photograph looks like an idyllic portrait of the American family: a mother, a father, and their two-year-old son.

But five years after that moment was captured on film, a new reality took hold: a savagely murdered mother, a quickly accused father, and a virtually orphaned son. That was how residents of Cleveland, Ohio, and eventually the nation, saw the Sheppard family in 1954. There was Marilyn Sheppard, a thirty-one-year-old, pregnant murder victim. There was Dr. Sam Sheppard, a thirty-year-old accused killer. And there was Sam Reese Sheppard, the seven-year-old boy who slept through his mother's murder.

What happened in the Sheppard home on the shores of Lake Erie on July 4, 1954, and what has followed in the decades since have been seared in the national consciousness. Few have not heard at least the basics of the story: Sam Sheppard, the handsome osteopathic surgeon, was charged with killing his wife, despite his assertions that the real culprit was a "bushy-haired" intruder with whom he fought twice during the incident. Under intense media coverage, Dr. Sheppard was convicted of the murder in what was then called "the trial of the century." A television series inspired by the case, *The Fugitive*, was popular in the 1960s and gave a very sympathetic portrayal of the father. Later, a movie of the same name, starring Harrison Ford and based loosely on the same story, was released.

The U.S. Supreme Court reversed Dr. Sheppard's conviction in 1966 on grounds that he did not receive a fair trial because of the pervasive publicity and news coverage. He was acquitted at his second trial that same year.

But Dr. Sheppard was never able to escape the shame and suspicion that followed him. He died of liver failure at the age of forty-six in 1970, a free but broken man. All the while, Sam Reese Sheppard never believed that his father killed his mother. More than forty years after that Independence Day that had changed his life, Sam Reese Sheppard coauthored a book containing new information about the case, which raised questions about another man's likely involvement. Several months after the book was published in 1995, an attorney for the Sheppard family, Terry Gilbert, filed a petition in Cuyahoga County, Ohio, asking that Dr. Sheppard be declared innocent of his wife's murder. It was an unusual distinction, peculiar to Ohio law, that required Gilbert to go beyond proving Dr. Sheppard was "not guilty," to proving him "innocent." If they could get that ruling, it would open the door for them to pursue monetary damages for wrongful imprisonment.

It was at the beginning of this new legal battle, which I eventually joined, that some surprising facts were revealed that convinced me of the real killer's probable identity. By the time I started working on the case in early 1998, much had already happened, and I spent a good deal of time getting up to speed by reviewing trial transcripts and other official records that Gilbert sent me.

●　•　●

In the summer of 1954, I had finished my second year of medical school and was working in Pittsburgh as a camp counselor at a day camp. I heard about the Sheppard murder, but didn't give it much thought other than the fact that it was a doctor's wife. I followed it a bit more closely when the U.S. Supreme Court granted Dr. Sheppard a new trial, and took notice of the work done by his attorney at the time, F. Lee Bailey. I later became friends with Bailey and worked with him over the years on many, many cases.

The materials I now had from Terry Gilbert provided much more detail about the events before and after Marilyn Sheppard's bludgeoning death.

The night of July 3, 1954, the Sheppards had their neighbors, Don and Nancy Ahern, over for dinner at their home in Bay Village, an affluent suburb of Cleveland. The two couples enjoyed the evening and watched television after eating. Dr. Sheppard, who had worked a shift at Bay View Hospital that day, stretched out on a day bed and eventually fell asleep. The Aherns left and Marilyn Sheppard, four months pregnant with a boy, went upstairs to their bedroom. Dr. Sheppard later recalled being awakened in the early morning hours by his wife's cries.

He rushed up the stairs to find out what was happening, but Dr. Sheppard said he quickly was knocked unconscious by a blow from behind. When he awoke, he heard a noise downstairs and went to investigate. That was when he saw the dark figure of a man and chased him down a long set of stairs toward the lake. Another struggle ensued on the beach before Dr. Sheppard was again knocked out on the shore of Lake Erie. After regaining consciousness a second time, he returned to the house and found his wife dead.

About twenty minutes before 6 A.M., Dr. Sheppard called his friend and neighbor, Spencer Houk, who also was mayor of Bay Village. "My God, Spen, get over here quick! I think they've killed Marilyn!"[1] Houk and his wife, Esther, soon arrived, followed by police; Dr. Sheppard's brother, Dr. Richard Sheppard; and others. That included members of the press, who were given access to the house. The coroner of Cuyahoga County, Dr. Samuel Gerber, got to the scene at about 7:50 A.M. and entered the Sheppards' bedroom roughly ten minutes later. Marilyn Sheppard and the bed she was on were a bloody mess.

She was lying face up with her head resting in about the middle of the bed and turned slightly to the right. Her legs dangled over the end of the bed, and a bunched up sheet covered the lower part of her body. Her pajama top was pushed up, exposing her breasts and abdomen, while her pajama bottoms had been removed from one leg. Marilyn Sheppard's face and head were covered in blood, and a large area of the bed was stained as well. Blood had splattered on a pillow at the head of the bed and a closet door to the right.

A trail of blood also ran from the bedroom, down the stairs and out the door toward the lake. Investigators theorized that this was Marilyn Sheppard's blood, which had dripped from the weapon used in the assault as her killer made an exit. Local Bay Village police as well as officers from the Cleveland police department investigated the scene, but it was hardly secured. Newspaper photographers were allowed inside, even into the room that still contained Marilyn Sheppard's beaten body.[2]

Signs of a disturbance were elsewhere in the house. Several drawers were pulled out of a desk in the den. Near the desk, investigators found a wrench, a screwdriver, and several other tools, along with a bloodstained watch that belonged to Marilyn Sheppard. Outside the house, a green bag was found and inside it was a chain, some keys, a ring, and another watch with blood on it. This one belonged to Dr. Sheppard.

Dr. Gerber, meanwhile, prepared to interview Dr. Sheppard, who had been taken by his brother to Bay View Hospital to be treated for a fractured vertebra in his neck and other bruises. But before Dr. Gerber left the house, he told investigators, "Well, it is evident the doctor did this, so let's go get the confession out of him."[3] At the hospital, Dr. Gerber questioned Dr. Sheppard, who had been sedated with a painkiller. Dr. Sheppard had a large bruise on the right side of his face near his eye, but neither the coroner nor anyone else who examined Dr. Sheppard found any open wounds. Dr. Gerber also collected the water-soaked clothing Dr. Sheppard had been wearing. There was a spot of blood near the knee of his right pant leg, but no other bloodstains could be found on the rest of his clothes.

More detectives arrived at Dr. Sheppard's hospital bed later in the day with more questions. He spoke to Det. Robert Schottke and his partner, answering their inquiries as best he could. At the end of the interview, Schottke told Dr. Sheppard, "I think you killed your wife."

Back at the house, Dr. Gerber returned to the bedroom. At about 10:30 A.M., he examined Marilyn Sheppard's body and concluded that rigor mortis, or body stiffening, had "set in." I inferred the coroner meant "fixed." Dr. Gerber also noted that lividity, or blood pooling, was present on her body; however, he did not indicate whether it was fixed. Based on that information, as well as the later autopsy report and statements from the Aherns, the coroner estimated Marilyn Sheppard died between 3 A.M. and 4 A.M.

Once her body was removed from the bed, Dr. Gerber found parts of two teeth in the bedding. Although the coroner initially did not believe they were from Marilyn Sheppard, it later was established they indeed had come from her mouth. Dr. Gerber also looked at the pillow found at the head of the bed. One side had blood spatter on it. The other was soaked with blood, except for the outline of what he believed was a surgical instrument. He described the instrument, based on the outline, as having two blades that were each three inches long and with teethlike indentations at the tips. There was a space between the blades. Dr. Gerber later said a medical instrument was the weapon used to batter Marilyn Sheppard, although authorities could never find one like the one he described.

Dr. Gerber, who was not a pathologist, did not perform the autopsy. It was conducted by his chief deputy, Dr. Lester Adelson, an experienced and respected forensic pathologist. After cleaning the abundant dried blood from Marilyn Sheppard's head, face, neck, and hands, Dr. Adelson documented extensive injuries. He counted fifteen lacerations, or cuts, on her forehead and scalp. Some were gaping, some crescentic (crescent shaped). They ranged in size from a half inch by a quarter inch to two and a quarter inches by a half inch. Many were so severe they extended down to the skull bone. Both eyes were swollen, her nose was fractured, and a small abrasion was found on the bridge of her nose.

Dr. Adelson also found that parts of two teeth—the upper right and left medial incisors—were missing, with a laceration/contusion of the adjacent inner upper lip. A contusion, or bruise, that was two inches in diameter was located on her right shoulder, and there were multiple abrasions on her right forearm and hand. A joint on the pinky finger of her right hand showed hypermobility, which meant it was likely dislocated or broken. On her left forearm was a contused abrasion, or bruise in which the skin was also scraped, and the nail of the fourth finger on her left hand was partially avulsed, or torn away: all were indications to me that Marilyn Sheppard tried to fight her attacker and ward off the blows.

When Dr. Adelson pulled back the scalp, he found extensive hemorrhaging. The fractures of the frontal bone were severely "comminuted," which meant the bone was pulverized and displaced. Dr. Adelson noted he could easily pick small fragments of bone from those areas. Although there was no epidural hemorrhaging—bleeding on the outside of the brain's protective covering called the dura—there was plenty of hemorrhaging subdurally, or beneath the dura. On each side of the brain in that area there was twenty ccs (cubic centimeters) of blood, about five teaspoons' worth. Dr. Adelson also documented more hemorrhaging and bruising throughout other parts of the brain. The fact that there was plenty of blood was an indication that Marilyn Sheppard was alive and her heart was beating for at least a short time after she suffered her injuries.

An external exam of Marilyn Sheppard's vagina revealed it to be of "a normal female," according to Dr. Adelson. Internally, he found a moderate amount of "creamy white exudate," which is simply a viscous discharge that could be related to bacteria or fungus. When he looked under a microscope at swabbings taken from her vagina, Dr. Adelson saw abundant epithelial cells—cells that line internal body tissues, including the vagina—and bacteria. He found no spermatozoa or other indications that she had been sexually assaulted.

In all, Dr. Adelson documented thirty-five separate injuries to Marilyn Sheppard. He listed the cause of death as the multiple blows to her head and face, the skull fractures, and the brain hemorrhages and contusions. The manner was "homicide by assault."

●•●

From the beginning, the murder drew intense media interest. Within days, the stories and headlines took on accusatory tones based on information—some of it inaccurate—given by the authorities. Officials had complained Dr. Sheppard wouldn't talk to them, and headlines repeatedly stressed his lack of cooperation. "Testify Now in Death, Bay Doctor Is Ordered," was one headline. (In fact, he had spoken with them on several occasions.) Another, over a front-page editorial calling for Dr. Sheppard's arrest, said, "Somebody Is Getting Away with Murder." On July 21, 1954, another front-page editorial called for Dr. Gerber to convene an inquest. Later that day, he did.

The three-day event, held in a local school gymnasium to accommodate the press and other interested crowds, began the next day. A coroner's inquest then, as now, is much like a preliminary hearing in cases. As the elected coroner of Allegheny County, I have held inquests in the past. During some, detectives present their evidence and the coroner determines whether a suspect should be held over for action by prosecutors. But the coroner doesn't have the power to charge someone with a crime. I should note that in conducting inquests in highly controversial cases, I always use an attorney—my solicitor—to conduct the hearings, with my input when necessary. In the Sheppard case, Dr. Gerber ran the show. He issued a subpoena to Dr. Sheppard, who testified for many hours, although his attorney was not permitted to take part or introduce evidence. (Defense attorneys are not entitled to participate in inquests, although in my office I allow them to as a courtesy.) During his testimony, Dr. Sheppard was asked whether he had had an extramarital affair. He lied and said no, which was used against him at trial when prosecutors brought in his lover.

After the conclusion of the inquest, Dr. Gerber issued what is known as a coroner's verdict. "The injuries that caused this death were inflicted by her husband," he wrote. As support, the coroner said it was impossible to believe Dr. Sheppard's explanation. He noted that Dr. Sheppard never fully cooperated with police and pointed out that he had called two lawyers sometime on July 4 or 5.[4]

Authorities arrested Dr. Sheppard on July 30, 1954, and a grand jury indicted him on murder charges August 17. His first trial began with jury selection on October 18. By then, all the prospective jurors' names had been published in the newspapers, and all of them received anonymous calls or letters, or calls from friends, about the case before they had even gone to court. Dozens of reporters sat in on the trial, and many were given seats inside the bar, the area of the courtroom generally restricted to lawyers, court personnel, and other trial participants.

The trial continued for eight weeks, during which Dr. Sheppard testified in his defense, denying that he had killed his wife. Jurors deliberated for five days before finding Dr. Sheppard guilty of second-degree murder. He was sentenced to life in prison. There were appeals and rejections until 1964, when a federal district court judge ruled Dr. Sheppard was not given a fair trial. Two years later, in June 1966, the U.S. Supreme Court agreed with the district court ruling and ordered that Dr. Sheppard receive a new trial.

"The fact is that bedlam reigned at the courthouse during the [first] trial and newsmen took over practically the entire courtroom, hounding most of the participants in the trial, especially Sheppard," the Supreme Court wrote in its opinion, at one point calling the proceedings a "carnival."

The second trial did not last nearly as long as the first, and on November 16, 1966, jurors found Dr. Sheppard not guilty. This case was a major touchstone in the early part of attorney F. Lee Bailey's stellar career as a criminal defense lawyer.

●•●

The wrongful-imprisonment lawsuit that had been filed by attorney Terry Gilbert in 1995 sought to have Dr. Sheppard declared "innocent"—a much higher legal hurdle to overcome than just a finding of "not guilty." But to do that, there had to be strong evidence that someone else had killed Marilyn Sheppard. That's where Richard Eberling came into the picture.

Back in November 1959, police arrested Eberling for burglarizing homes in Cleveland. Authorities searched his home and found two rings that had belonged to Marilyn Sheppard, including her engagement ring. Eberling told police he stole the rings from the home of Dr. Richard Sheppard, Dr. Sam Sheppard's brother. He also told police he washed windows at Sam Sheppard's house and was there several days before the murder. Unprompted, he said he was working at the house when he cut his finger on a kitchen window and bled throughout the residence.

Detectives questioned him further about Marilyn Sheppard's murder and even gave him a polygraph examination later in the month. The examiner believed Eberling passed, and although questions later were raised about how accurately the results were interpreted, police lost interest in the burglar. More than two decades later, detectives were again looking at Eberling's possible connection with another woman's death.

This time it was a ninety-year-old widow named Ethel Durkin, who lived in a suburb of Cleveland. Eberling had worked around Durkin's home since the late 1950s and acted as one of her caretakers for several years before her death. Durkin supposedly suffered a fall at her house in November 1983 and died at a hospital two months later. Her death initially was ruled an accident, but the case was declared a homicide in 1988 after more investigation. Eberling was charged with aggravated murder and various counts of grand theft after authorities uncovered a scheme by him to swindle money from Durkin's estate. In July 1989, a jury convicted Eberling of aggravated murder, theft, and forgery, and he was sentenced to life in prison.

Though the authorities did not seem interested in Richard Eberling as a suspect in the murder of Marilyn Sheppard, others were. While researching his book in the late eighties and early nineties, Sam Reese Sheppard and his coauthor, Cynthia Cooper, spoke to a man who said he had worked for Eberling's window-washing business in the fifties. The man, Lavern "Vern" Lund, said that he had worked alone at the Sheppard house July 2, 1954, two days before Marilyn Sheppard was killed. That was significant because Eberling had told police in 1959 that he cut his finger while working at the Sheppard residence just a few days before the murder. If Lund was telling the truth, then when did Eberling bleed in the house?

For years, however, the question of whose blood was in the bedroom and where the trail of blood leading out of the house came from had gone unanswered. In the days and weeks after Marilyn Sheppard's murder, many pieces of bloodstained evidence were examined by the Cuyahoga County coroner's office. In those days, investigators didn't have the advanced testing capabilities available today, but they were able to group human blood or bloodstains into four types—A, B, AB, or O. A sample of Marilyn Sheppard's blood showed it to be type O. The only bloodstained item technicians typed was the bedsheet on which she was lying. It also was type O.

However, aside from determining that the blood trail was from a human, no typing was done. The same was true for blood found on watches that belonged to Marilyn and Sam Sheppard, and blood spatters found on the bedroom wall. In fact, some of the most comprehensive crime scene analysis was done, not by police, the coroner's office, or any state agency, but by a criminalist hired by the Sheppard family after Dr. Sheppard's conviction in 1954. A criminalist examines such things as tire tracks or hidden bloodstains, as well as trace evidence such as DNA or fibers, to help solve crimes.

Dr. Paul Kirk was a professor of biochemistry and criminalistics at the University of California, and a pioneer in the use of forensic science to decipher crime scenes. He spent two days in

January 1955 examining the room where Marilyn Sheppard was killed and the rest of the house, conducting a detailed analysis of the blood spatter patterns. Dr. Kirk found blood spots on every wall of the bedroom, but not evenly distributed. Large amounts of blood spatter were on the wall to Marilyn Sheppard's right, or the east wall, which also included a closet door.

What Dr. Kirk found interesting about some of the blood spots on that wall was that they contrasted with the spatter found elsewhere. While spots throughout the rest of the room were considered high-velocity spatter—that is, the blood was traveling very quickly when it made impact—the ones on the east wall were low-velocity drops. Most of them hit the surface at nearly right angles, which could be determined by their essentially round shape. Dr. Kirk concluded those blood spots must have been thrown off the murder weapon during its backswing. Based on that and other interpretations of the blood spatter patterns, he also deduced the attacker must have used his left hand to deliver the blows.

In particular, one spot on the closet door on the east wall caught Dr. Kirk's attention. It was about one inch in diameter and nearly round, with no beading. Its characteristics meant the spot could not have come from impact spatter, or blood flying from a wound just after impact from a weapon. It also was not likely that the spot was thrown off a weapon. The most probable source was from a bleeding hand, Dr. Kirk decided, and not when that hand was wielding a weapon.

On the north wall, the one facing the foot of the bed, there were more high-velocity blood spots (identifiable by beading around the spot's periphery) in certain sections. But in an area in the corner where the north and east walls met there were no blood spots. Something must have blocked the blood's path, and Dr. Kirk believed he knew what it was—the body of Marilyn Sheppard's attacker. Based on the swath of clean wall, Dr. Kirk concluded the assailant must have stood near the foot of the bed on the east side. That meant the killer would have been covered in blood.

Dr. Kirk also went further than the state's investigators regarding typing of bloodstains. They determined that the blood on the sheet was type O, the same type as Marilyn Sheppard's. But when Dr. Kirk tested the large spot on the closet door that intrigued him, he found differences in the way the blood reacted compared to another spot on the wall and a stain on the mattress. For example, it was less soluble when mixed with distilled water. Although his tests indicated the stain was type O blood, Dr. Kirk believed the differences in the way it reacted during testing was proof enough that it came from someone other than Marilyn Sheppard.

Then there were the bloodstains on Dr. Sheppard's watch, which was found in a green bag outside the house. The band had been broken, and several bloodstains were noted on the surface of the watch crystal and in the links. Mary Cowan, a laboratory analyst at the coroner's office, had tried to type the blood but was unable to do so. Dr. Kirk deduced that the watchband appeared to have broken when someone else ripped it off Dr. Sheppard's wrist. "It is difficult to accept the idea that a person would remove his own watch so violently as to damage the band to the extent that exists," Dr. Kirk wrote in his April 1955 affidavit.[5] Cowan testified at the second trial that she thought the blood on the watch was spatter, what one would expect if an assailant was wearing the watch during an attack on Marilyn Sheppard. But Dr. Kirk said he believed the blood on the watch looked more like a smear, or it had been transferred by contact with something bloody.

Besides the bloodstains, the broken teeth interested Dr. Kirk. He noted in his report that prosecutors never bothered to explain why they were there. Had those teeth been fractured from a blow to her mouth, one would expect to see injuries to the lips as well. But those were not present. Dr. Kirk believed it was more likely the teeth were pulled outward because they were found outside Marilyn Sheppard's mouth and the fracture angle of one tooth was consistent with a pull outward. He theorized that Marilyn Sheppard bit her attacker's hand or finger and he yanked it violently from her mouth. That injury would likely bleed and would explain how a large, low-velocity blood spot could be deposited on the closet door.

Along with working on evidence in the bedroom, Dr. Kirk dealt with the blood trail through other parts of the house. He did not believe, as prosecutors had contended, that the stains came from the murder weapon dripping spots of Marilyn Sheppard's blood. To prove this, he conducted experiments with various instruments ranging from a wrench to a brass bar that he dipped in blood. Dr. Kirk recorded how long and how far it took for the blood to stop dripping from those objects. Almost all of them shed their drops within fifteen feet, and the drops were always small. In contrast, the blood trails found in the Sheppard house were larger. Dr. Kirk's conclusion: at least some of the blood trails came from an injury on the killer's body that was dripping blood. It was a significant issue, because Dr. Sheppard had no bleeding wounds on July 4, 1954.

Dr. Kirk's comprehensive review of the case also led him to conclude that the murder began as some sort of sexual assault and that the weapon used was likely a heavy, rounded object such as a flashlight.

In 1996, Sam Reese Sheppard and the others involved in the latest investigation of the case wanted to build upon Dr. Kirk's work. They needed a tool of science that wasn't available decades ago—DNA testing. They turned to Dr. Mohammad Tahir, one of the leading experts in DNA testing and the DNA technical manager at the Indianapolis-Marion County Forensic Services Agency in Indiana.

Dr. Tahir wanted to test known samples against bloodstains found at the crime scene and throughout the Sheppard house. Attorney Gilbert had gotten court permission to obtain a blood sample from Richard Eberling, so they had that standard. There also were some head hairs from Marilyn Sheppard. Direct DNA samples from Dr. Sheppard were not available, so Dr. Tahir tried to recover genetic material from stamps on letters Dr. Sheppard had sent to Marilyn in 1943 before they were married. The idea was that DNA from his saliva—deposited when he licked the stamps—might have been left on those items.

Other items Dr. Tahir tested were a stain from Marilyn Sheppard's bedsheet, two vaginal swabs, the bloodstain from Dr. Sheppard's pants, and a wood chip from the basement stairs of the house. Unfortunately, Dr. Tahir was able to recover only enough DNA from the stamps to obtain a partial genetic profile of Dr. Sheppard. He was, however, able to perform testing on the other items, and in early 1997 made two important findings.

One was that there definitely was a third person in the Sheppard house the night Marilyn Sheppard was killed, and that person could have been Eberling, but the testing was not more specific. Dr. Tahir discovered that the bloodstains found on the wood chip and on Dr. Sheppard's pants were not from Marilyn Sheppard. Even the police and prosecutors who believed Dr. Sheppard killed his wife acknowledged he had no open wounds immediately following her death. So despite the fact that Dr. Tahir was not able to obtain DNA material from Dr. Sheppard, the blood on those two items—the stairs and the pants—must have come from a third person.

Dr. Tahir's other startling finding was sperm in the vaginal swabs. In 1954, officials at the Cuyahoga County coroner's office had purportedly examined those swabbings microscopically, but made no mention of sperm. The DNA from those samples was a mixture, and Eberling could not be ruled out as a partial contributor. When Sam

135

Reeese Sheppard's legal team released the results in February 1997, the news made the front page in papers across the country.

But the DNA testing was not over. The fact that Dr. Sheppard's DNA could not be accurately compared against the samples was a considerable shortcoming. Sam Reese Sheppard agreed to have his father's body exhumed, so in September 1997, bone, tooth, and fingernail samples were collected from the remains of Dr. Sheppard. In addition, Dr. Tahir had another sample to test that had not been available previously—dried scrapings from the bloodstain on the bedroom closet door that Dr. Kirk believed had come from Marilyn Sheppard's killer.

The results this time were slightly more conclusive. Dr. Tahir was able to say that two bloodstains from the trail in the house (one from the basement stairs and one from the porch) did not come from Dr. Sheppard or Marilyn Sheppard. The scientist also excluded Dr. Sheppard as the source of the bloodstain on his pants and as a donor of DNA found in the sperm fraction on the vaginal swabs. That was further support of Dr. Sheppard's story about an intruder and the theory that Marilyn Sheppard was sexually assaulted. As for the stain from the bedroom closet, Dr. Tahir concluded in a report that it was a mixture and was "consistent with having originated from Marilyn Sheppard and Richard Eberling." He could not tell, because of limitations in the testing, whether Dr. Sheppard's DNA was present in the closet door stain. Further limiting the definitiveness of the results was the possibility of contamination over the decades.

Nonetheless, with the latest findings, attorney Terry Gilbert marshaled his forces and called a press conference on March 5, 1998. "We now have, in 1998, conclusive evidence that Dr. Sheppard did not kill his wife," Gilbert told reporters. "In spite of the fact that he was acquitted in a second trial, this community has never owned up to the possibility that a terrible injustice occurred."[6]

Later, he raised the Eberling connection. "The trail of blood could only have come from the killer," Gilbert said. "And Richard Eberling cannot be removed from the equation. It presents the kind of compelling case that people are prosecuted and even put on death row for, every day in American courts."

Gilbert had asked me to consider several issues, among them whether the murder scene was processed properly and whether the injuries to Marilyn Sheppard were consistent with a sharp surgical instrument. The first question wasn't hard to answer. From my perspective, the coroner's office and police detectives did not do a thorough forensic investigation of the scene or, by extension, a thorough medicolegal evaluation of the evidence.

I had come to a similar conclusion many years earlier when I reviewed a horrible shoot-out between authorities and a group of black nationalists in the Cleveland community known as Glenville. The death toll from the incident on July 23, 1968, stood at three police officers, three black nationalists, and one bystander. Fourteen others were wounded. The group's leader, Fred Ahmed Evans, was arrested on murder charges, and his attorneys asked me to consult with them.

Within weeks of the shootings, I traveled to Cleveland to examine the scene and went to the coroner's office to review the autopsy records, clothing of the victims, microscopic slides, and other materials. I first noted errors in the autopsy of a civilian, who had been shot in the head while supposedly driving a police officer into the line of fire to help recover wounded officers. The pathologist who examined the man described what clearly was a bullet entrance wound as an exit wound. Close-up photos of the injury also showed black powder deposits around it, an indication the man had been shot at very close range, what I would consider execution style.

As I inspected the other autopsy reports, including those of the police officers, I realized a critical part of each was missing—the toxicology test results. When I asked about them, the coroner's staff reluctantly retrieved them for me, and I soon learned why there may have been some hesitation. Two of the three dead officers had significant blood-alcohol levels. One had a blood alcohol level of 0.19 percent and the other a level of 0.25 percent. At the time in Ohio, a level of 0.15 percent was considered too drunk to drive. And these men had been on duty for six to eight hours when they were killed, so they either drank very heavily before arriving for work, or were drinking on the job. Either way, it didn't look good for the police and their version of how the black nationalists instigated the shoot-out.

I was shocked that the coroner's office had withheld that information from not only the defense attorneys, but also the public in general. To me, the incident was more than just sloppiness or negligence by the coroner's office. The coroner during both the Glenville shoot-out and the Sheppard murder was the same person: Dr. Samuel Gerber.

In the Sheppard case, I considered the position of Marilyn Sheppard's body as it was found on the bed and the condition of her pajamas. She was found with her head about a third of the way down the bed, and her legs were dangling over the foot of the bed, bent at the knees. Her legs were pushed apart. The pants of her pajamas had been removed from one leg and the pajama tops had been pushed up on her torso, exposing her breasts. The injuries described in the autopsy report and the ones I saw in many pictures were mainly blunt force trauma of the head and upper extremities. That wouldn't cause her pajama bottoms to somehow come off of one leg.

The scene clearly suggested some sort of sexual assault to me. Yet as far as I could tell, there was no indication that either the coroner, Dr. Samuel Gerber, or Dr. Adelson, who performed the autopsy, seriously considered such a possibility. During his examination, Dr. Adelson summed up his findings of the area around Marilyn Sheppard's vagina in six words: "The external genitalia are normal female." In my opinion, the pathologist should have conducted a careful and detailed rape study. Swabs from the mouth, vagina, and anus should have been taken at the scene. Dr. Adelson did take vaginal swabs, but there was no record that showed testing of the other areas was done. Additionally, Dr. Adelson noted that the swabs he took and made into slides exhibited no indications of sperm. However, when Dr. Tahir examined the same slides more than forty years later, he found sperm heads.

I also took issue with the way Dr. Gerber dealt with the teeth fragments found when moving Marilyn Sheppard's body from the bed. He initially believed—wrongly, as it turned out—that the fragments came from her attacker and not her. Dr. Adelson found clear evidence during the autopsy that the teeth fragments did indeed come from Marilyn Sheppard, but neither he nor Dr. Gerber made any sort of conclusion as to how they were broken off. The coroner also, as far as I could tell, didn't consult with a forensic odontologist or forensic dentist. But the new team pursuing the wrongful-imprisonment case against the state of Ohio did.

Dr. Michael Sobel, a forensic odontologist from Pittsburgh, whom I know quite well and who has been a longtime consultant for the Allegheny County coroner's office, also worked on the case for Sam Reese Sheppard. He came to a conclusion (the same one I had reached) that differed from Dr. Kirk's interpretation of Marilyn Sheppard's teeth injuries. Dr. Kirk believed Marilyn Sheppard must have bitten her attacker and lost part of two teeth through that method. It was a reasonable argument. But I felt the more likely scenario was that those injuries occurred through blunt force trauma. Part of Dr. Kirk's theory was based on the fact there were no surrounding injuries to her mouth or face, but the autopsy did note a crusted abrasion, or scrape, on the inside of Marilyn Sheppard's lower lip. Dr. Sobel and I believed it was more likely that she was struck in the face, causing the fractures. Dr. Sobel noted that during a violent struggle, a person's lips often are pulled back, which would have exposed the teeth to potential damage without significant injuries to the lips.

Another part of Dr. Kirk's analysis that diverged from both Dr. Sobel's and my interpretation of the evidence dealt with how Marilyn Sheppard may have injured her attacker, causing him to bleed. While Dr. Kirk theorized that she bit her assailant, Dr. Sobel and I were able to consider facts Dr. Kirk did not have available to him in 1955 relating to Richard Eberling. First there were the DNA tests. While they were not discriminatory to the exclusion of all others, the results could not rule out Eberling as a contributor to genetic material found in the Sheppard house. Further suspicion was cast upon Eberling when a former nurse of the woman he was convicted of killing said in 1996 that he had confessed to murdering Marilyn Sheppard many years earlier. And one of Eberling's fellow inmates claimed that in early 1998 Eberling acknowledged raping and killing Dr. Sheppard's wife.

However, Eberling denied making the confessions and continued to say he was not involved in Marilyn Sheppard's death, until his death in July 1998 at sixty-eight. But Eberling's death may have helped the reinvestigation of the crime in a small way. An autopsy revealed a half-inch scar on the inside of his left wrist. When police arrested Eberling in 1959 for burglarizing homes, they described a similar scar on his left wrist. How did it get there? Dr. Kirk believed Marilyn Sheppard would have left a bite mark on her killer's hand or arm.

Dr. Sobel, however, looked at autopsy pictures of the scar and concluded it did not look like a bite mark. He considered it to be more of a gouge or deep scratch. That fit quite nicely with another injury to Marilyn Sheppard that the initial investigators seemed to give little consideration—the partially avulsed (torn) fingernail on the fourth finger of her left hand. It was entirely plausible to believe that while fighting for her life, Marilyn Sheppard dug her nail into her attacker's wrist or scratched him, partially tearing it while at the same time causing a bleeding wound to her assailant. Had Dr. Gerber considered such a scenario, perhaps the need to type all of the blood found in the house would have been clearer.

I believe that the investigation suffered mightily from Dr. Gerber's premature conclusion that Dr. Sheppard killed his wife. If the forensic lapses that followed had been avoided, there was a good chance more information corroborating Dr. Sheppard's story of an intruder could have been developed. Instead, the blood trail went untested for decades. The blood spatter in the bedroom also was assumed to have originated only from Marilyn Sheppard, a conclusion Dr. Kirk showed was faulty by his work less than a year after the murder.

Beyond the issue of consulting a forensic odontologist, however, I felt there were other lapses in the way Dr. Gerber approached the crime scene. While the experience I have gained from conducting or reviewing tens of thousands of autopsies is invaluable, I realize there are some areas in which others have more expertise. There are specialists skilled in specific areas, such as blood spatter and other areas of forensic science, whom I call upon to help me in my investigations. Dr. Gerber, who was not trained as a forensic pathologist, did not appear to have done that. From what I could discern from the reports, the coroner's office criminalist didn't even go to the scene. The only materials that were examined were those items Dr. Gerber personally deemed to be important.

One of the other issues Terry Gilbert asked me to review was whether Marilyn Sheppard's wounds were consistent with a surgical instrument of some kind. Again, my short answer was no. The wounds to her head were clearly caused by blunt force trauma rather than sharp instrument trauma. Had a sharp instrument been used, there would have been incisions or stab wounds, and Dr. Adelson, who performed the autopsy, described no such injuries. Instead, he found several lacerations, or cuts, that were crescentic, or slightly curved.

Sharp instruments generally don't leave crescentic lacerations. Cylindrical objects do. I believed something like a pipe or a flashlight could have caused all the wounds found on Marilyn Sheppard. Dr. Kirk had come to the same conclusion forty-four years earlier, and once again, it was prior to evidentiary revelations in the case that tended to support the theory. In August 1955, the Sheppards' next-door neighbor found something while swimming in Lake Erie, not thirty feet from the Sheppards' property line. It was a flashlight. The neighbor, Karl Schuele, told police he discovered the three-cell flashlight in about eighteen inches of water. Bay Village police chief John Eaton wrote in a report that "the light has been damaged by striking something repeatedly and the case has been dented on the side about where a person's thumb would come."

The chief turned his report over to Cleveland homicide detectives, and the flashlight made its way to the coroner's office. But Dr. Gerber apparently did little or nothing with the instrument. As far as I could determine, no testing or forensic examination of the flashlight for trace evidence was ever done, and it later was discarded. There was little likelihood any blood would have remained on the flashlight, since it had been submerged for what Chief Eaton considered "some time." However, the damaged casing could have been and should have been tested for tissues or hairs that might have become embedded in it during an attack.

＊ ＊ ＊

But as Gilbert and his team continued to push forward for another trial—to have Dr. Sheppard declared innocent—prosecutors continued to fight against the civil lawsuit and sought to have it dismissed. The state argued that Dr. Sheppard's right to sue ended with his death. The battle reached the Ohio Supreme Court, which decided in December 1998 to allow the wrongful-imprisonment suit to move forward. As part of their defense of the case, prosecutors wanted to disinter Marilyn Sheppard's body and that of her fetus from a crypt in suburban Cleveland. Officials said publicly they wanted to obtain new DNA samples and reexamine her wounds. Privately, prosecutors wanted to obtain DNA from the fetus to see if Dr. Sheppard really was the father. If he wasn't, the argument could be made that Dr. Sheppard killed his wife in a rage after discovering such a fact.[7] I thought that the whole idea was rotten, and I later learned DNA testing showed 99.99 percent certainty that Dr. Sheppard was the father.[8]

I was present, as were many others, when her remains were removed on October 5, 1999. Along with a large contingent of media, Gilbert and the other experts working with him were there, as well as members of the prosecutor's office and the coroner's office. What remained of Marilyn Sheppard's body was transported to the coroner's office, where x-rays were taken of her skull and genetic samples retrieved. I and the other forensic pathologists and scientists inspected the mostly skeletalized remains, but there was nothing new to learn from them.

Still, Cuyahoga County officials refused to concede the possibility that Dr. Sheppard was innocent of killing his wife. Faced with what I considered substantial evidence pointing to another assailant, prosecutors tried to find ways to shoot down the material and theories presented by Gilbert and his team. They also clung to Dr. Gerber's speculation that the murder weapon was a sharp instrument. One of the things the state did was consult with C. Owen Lovejoy, Ph.D., an anthropology professor from Kent State University, who conducted a head injury reconstruction to determine the patterns left by various instruments ranging from a 1950s-style flashlight to an adjustable wrench.

Dr. Lovejoy used a skull, clay as soft tissue, and enamel as a sort of outer layer to simulate Marilyn Sheppard's head. He then employed a dowel to act as the spinal column and used a sand bag that weighed about seventy-five pounds for a human trunk. The entire setup was put on a mattress. After each blow, Dr. Lovejoy x-rayed the skull and examined the injuries. He struck the skull three times with the flashlight, but reported he was unable to fracture the skull and succeeded in causing only a laceration. Next came a pair of pliers for one blow, a fireplace poker for one blow, and a heavy adjustable wrench for two blows—each from a different position. Each of those strikes caused varying degrees of fractures or trauma.

While he concluded that Marilyn Sheppard's injuries were caused by blunt force trauma, he believed that the weapon was of a weight similar to that of the Channel Lock brand pliers. The flashlight, which Dr. Lovejoy said dented when he used it to strike the test skull, was probably too light. He also looked at autopsy photographs of Marilyn Sheppard's head injuries and noted what he considered flaking of the external cortex, which is the outer layer of the skull. The skull has two layers, or tables, of bone: the external cortex, which is thick and tough, and the layer underneath, which is thin, dense, and brittle.

The flaking that Dr. Lovejoy said he viewed exposed the diploe—a central layer of spongy bone between the skull's outer and inner layers—in two areas of the left parietal bone. The parietal bone is simply a portion of the skull, which is divided for medical purposes into many regions. The frontal area is located as it sounds, at the front of the head. The occipital region is at the back of the head, and the temporal sections are around the ears. The parietal area makes up the other parts of the skull.

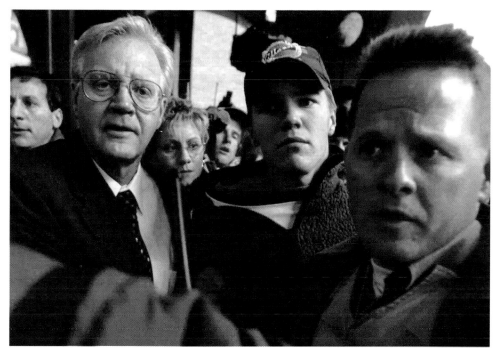

Brian Peterson, in ball cap, had to push his way through reporters to surrender to authorities on November 21, 1996. (Photo courtesy Chris Faytok/*The Star-Ledger*.)

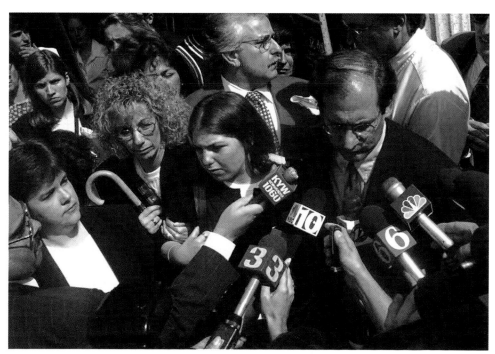

Amy Grossberg and her attorney, Robert Gottlieb, are surrounded by the media on July 3, 1997, in Wilmington, Delaware. (Photo courtesy John O'Boyle/*The Star-Ledger*.)

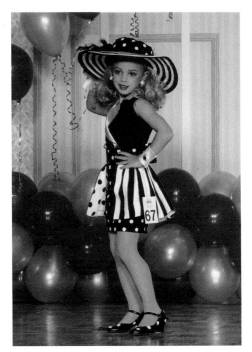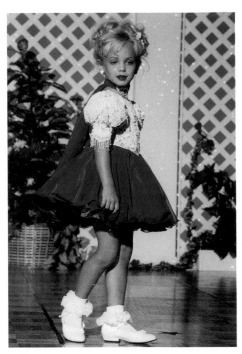

JonBenet Ramsey wore extravagant and very adult outfits while participating in beauty pageants. (Photo courtesy Mark Fix/Zuma Press Inc.)

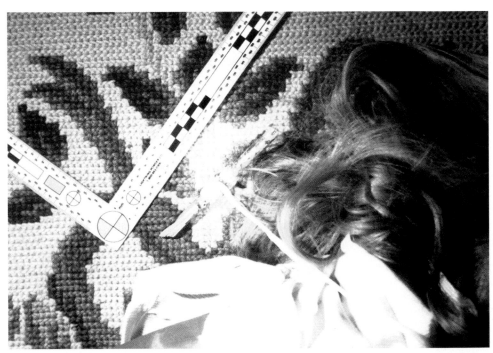

The rope and stick used to fashion a ligature around JonBenet Ramsey's neck are visible. (Photo courtesy Dr. Henry Lee.)

The mark near Ted Binion's solar plexus could not have been caused by someone sitting on him, as prosecutors alleged, because of the concave shape of his chest. (Photo courtesy Dr. Michael Baden.)

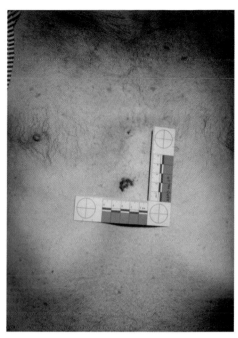

A closer look at the mark, which is shaped like a shirt button. (Photo courtesy Dr. Michael Baden.)

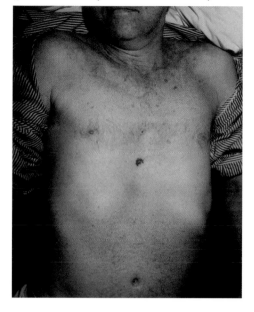

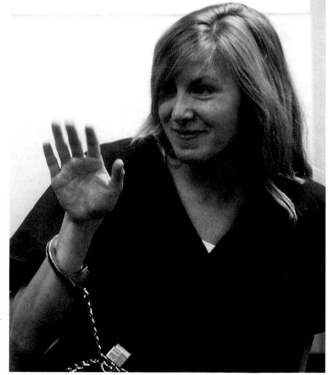

Binion's girlfriend, Sandy Murphy, waves to her parents at her arraignment on June 29, 1999. (Photo courtesy AP/ Wide World Photos.)

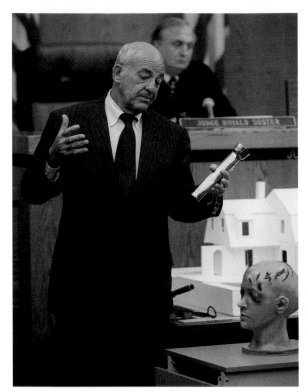

Dr. Cyril Wecht testifies in February 2000 during the civil trial brought by Sam Reese Sheppard to have his father, Dr. Sam Sheppard, declared innocent of his wife's 1954 murder. (Photo courtesy David Andersen/ *The Plain Dealer*.)

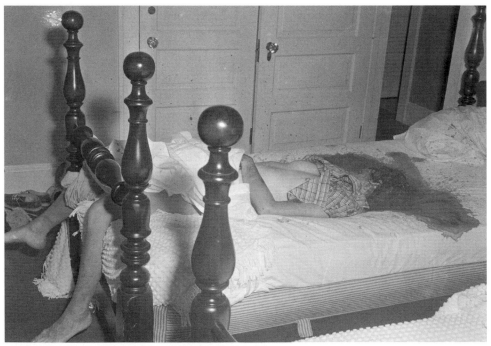

Blood stains on the bed and walls of Marilyn Sheppard's bedroom provided important clues about the crime. (Photo introduced into evidence during original Sheppard trial.)

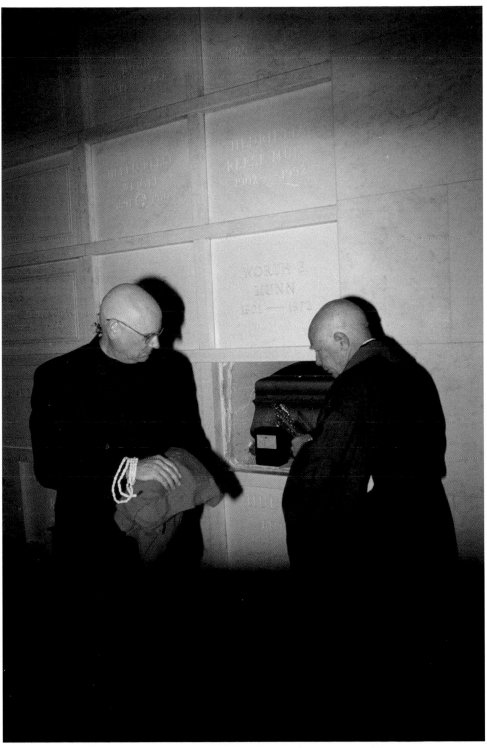

Sam Reese Sheppard and a monk at the crypt that held his mother's remains prior to her coffin being disinterred in October 1999. (Photo courtesy Dr. Michael Sobel.)

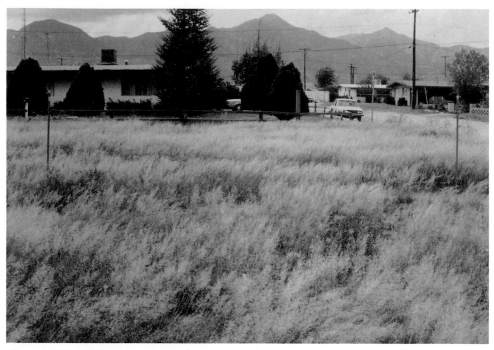

The gun battle that occurred in this field in Miracle Valley, Arizona, left two religious sect members dead. (Photo courtesy Dr. Cyril Wecht.)

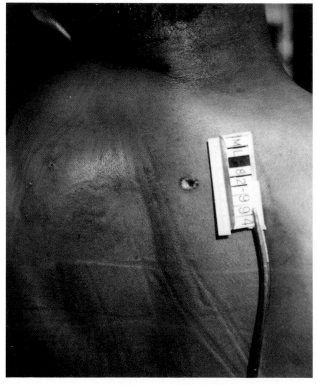

The bullet hole in William Thomas Jr.'s lower left back is an entrance wound. (Photo courtesy Dr. Cyril Wecht.)

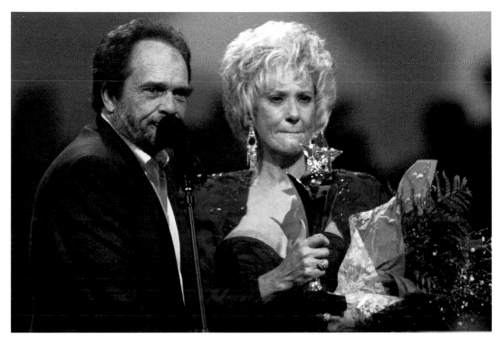

Tammy Wynette, known as the first lady of country music, received the living legend award from Merle Haggard at the TNN Music City News Country Awards in Nashville, Tennessee, on June 10, 1991. (Photo courtesy AP/Wide World Photos.)

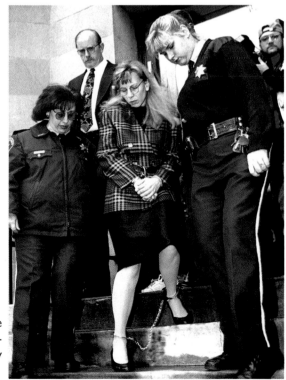

Joann Curley leaves the Luzerne County Courthouse after a bail hearing in December 1996. (Photo courtesy *Citizens' Voice*, Wilkes-Barre, Pa.)

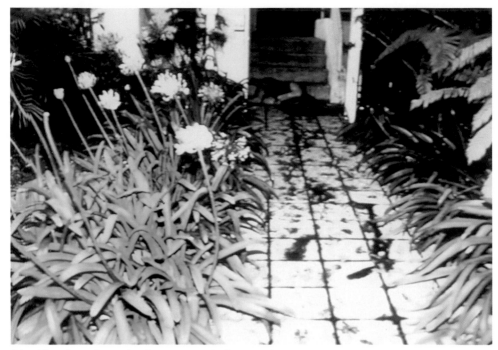

The bloody walkway leading to Nicole Simpson's condominium. Her body is in the background. (Photo courtesy Dr. Henry Lee.)

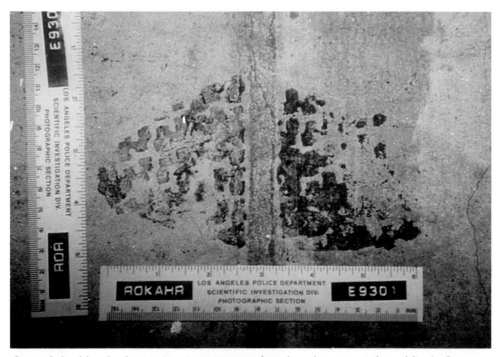

One of the bloody shoe prints investigators found at the scene where Nicole Simpson and Ron Goldman were murdered. (Photo courtesy Dr. Henry Lee.)

Those injuries, Dr. Lovejoy concluded, most likely were caused by a weapon with a sharp or ridged surface, and which had what he described as multiple "complex" surfaces.

First of all, I disagreed with his methodology of using the materials he did for testing purposes. Clay and enamel simply are not the equivalent of soft tissue and skin. Second, Dr. Lovejoy produced just one or two blows with a specific instrument before making his findings. The autopsy report and photos, however, document at least fifteen separate wounds to Marilyn Sheppard's head. I didn't think that his conclusions were reliable because he didn't accurately reproduce the attack.

I also took issue with Dr. Lovejoy's opinion about the likelihood that a sharp or ridged instrument had to have caused the "flaking" found on certain parts of Marilyn Sheppard's outer skull bone. I agreed with Dr. Lovejoy, however, that the injuries came from blunt force trauma. By its very nature, that kind of trauma is caused by blunt objects with a flat or rounded surface, not sharp ones. Additionally, what he referred to as flaking is something that is not limited to sharp-instrument injuries. When a bone is fractured, anything can happen, including separation of the outer table from the spongy bone. That too can be called flaking and isn't representative of any specific force.

Another person who examined evidence for prosecutors was James Wentzel, who digitized several photographs, including ones of Dr. Sheppard's watch. Wentzel said he observed small circular and elliptical bloodstains that were consistent with high-velocity spatter. He believed stains of that size would not have traveled for more than three feet from their source, intimating that at least Dr. Sheppard's watch would have been in the room where Marilyn Sheppard was killed.

I looked at the watch evidence somewhat differently. I believed that the watch was removed from Dr. Sheppard after he was knocked unconscious the first time, when he responded to his wife's cries and entered his darkened bedroom. Blood likely was transferred to the watch when the killer tore it from Dr. Sheppard's wrist or at a later time. Either way, the inability to conduct proper blood typing meant no one could even say whose blood was on the watch.

Prosecutors also turned to Cuyahoga County's current coroner, Dr. Elizabeth Balraj. She received her training in forensic pathology under Dr. Adelson's direction and worked with him for fifteen years. Dr. Balraj defended her colleague's work in the Sheppard case, specifically regarding his examination of Marilyn Sheppard's pubic area. She asserted he was a thorough and meticulous forensic pathologist. I generally agreed about Dr. Adelson's qualifications but felt he did an incomplete job with the Marilyn Sheppard autopsy. In a case of this nature, it would have been proper to offer a more detailed discussion and description of her lower abdomen and pelvic region, the thighs, the buttocks, and the specific areas of the genitalia—the mons pubis, the vulva, the vaginal lips, the vaginal mucosa, and the perineum (the area between the vagina and anus). Dr. Balraj argued that if Dr. Adelson had observed an injury to those regions, he would have noted it. My point was that he didn't document his observations one way or the other, so we'll never know for sure. (Due to illness during the most recent case, Dr. Adelson could not offer further clarification.)

Dr. Balraj further believed that Marilyn Sheppard's murder did not involve a sexual assault because, among other reasons, there were no documented injuries to the genitalia. She also suggested that a sexual assault was unlikely because of the position in which Marilyn Sheppard's body was found. Her legs dangled from the foot of the four-post bed and were under a horizontal wooden railing at the foot of it. Dr. Balraj argued that a sexual assault was impractical in that position. While it's true that was the final position of Marilyn Sheppard's body, the crime itself was not a static situation. This was a dynamic scene: she was fighting for her life and her attacker was administering blow after blow. It is not possible to ascertain the relative positions of an attacker and his victim during a violent, ever-changing struggle just from where a victim finally comes to rest.

● ˙ ●

The civil trial began in Cleveland at the end of January 2000 with jury selection in the courtroom of Cuyahoga County Common Pleas Court judge Ronald Suster. Two weeks later, on February 14, both sides gave their opening statements. Terry Gilbert went first, laying out the DNA evidence and other details that suggested Richard Eberling was the most likely suspect. "We are here to prove once and for all that Dr. Sheppard was innocent of the murder of his wife," Gilbert said. He later added, "Sometimes things go very, very wrong and lives are ruined. When the state makes a mistake it should be held accountable."[9]

Prosecutors, who were in the unusual position of defending a case, hammered home the theory that the marriage between Marilyn and Sam Sheppard was an unhappy one filled with infidelity and rejection. "We don't know what lit the match, but something caused the powder keg of marital conflict to blow early on the morning of July 4, 1954," prosecutor William Mason said.[10] Another prosecutor minimized the blood trail in the house and cast aspersions on Dr. Sheppard's character for the way he lived in the years leading up to his death.

The first witness to take the stand was F. Lee Bailey, the defense attorney who successfully argued the case before the U.S. Supreme Court and then represented Dr. Sheppard in the second trial in 1966. Bailey was followed by several others, including Sam Reese Sheppard, a detective who worked on the homicide back in 1954, and the nurse who said Eberling confessed to her that he killed Marilyn Sheppard. On February 25, forensic psychiatrist Dr. Emanuel Tanay told jurors that he believed Marilyn Sheppard's murder was a sexual sadistic homicide committed by a sadistic killer—not by a husband. "This was not a kind of outbreak of rage associated with spousal homicide," Tanay said. "This was sadistic rage. This was a sadistic orgy."[11]

Dr. Tanay, who had forty years of experience and once interviewed serial killer Ted Bundy, agreed with me that the murder clearly was sexually motivated. He looked to the same signs I did as indications of some sort of sexually related act—exposed breasts, legs spread, pajama bottoms halfway off. Part of Dr. Tanay's testimony was proffered outside the presence of the jury because of prosecutors' objections to it. The comments related to his opinion that Eberling was the kind of person who could have committed the crime, but Dr. Sheppard was not.

"That Dr. Sheppard was motivated to kill his wife and that he proceeded to kill her in this sadistic, brutal manner, and then did a cover-up, that whole thing, psychologically, in my opinion, makes no sense," Dr. Tanay said while jurors were out of the courtroom. "Dr. Sheppard is a most unlikely perpetrator of this type of sadistic homicide."[12]

Judge Suster did not permit jurors to hear those particular statements. By the time Dr. Tanay was done on the stand, it was the end of the second week of testimony. My turn was coming up the following Monday. I already had answered questions from one of the prosecutors, Steve Dever, who, along with Terry Gilbert, came to Pittsburgh one day in January to take my deposition.

Dever asked me then about my criticisms regarding the way the crime scene was handled.

"This was a death that literally cried out for the immediate presence of criminalists, whoever they would have been in Cuyahoga

County at that time—the police crime lab, state police crime lab, the coroner's office, whoever," I responded. "Such a scene just seemed to come from the pages of a textbook in a classroom—bloodstains here, blood spatters there, and the body. So I have a very strong criticism and truly great amazement that such people were not called by Dr. Gerber at that time.

"Dr. Gerber was not a criminalist. Forensic pathologists are not criminalists. We come to learn some things, but we are not trained criminalists. And especially since Dr. Gerber had no training as a forensic pathologist, that deficiency was even greater and more relevant."

When I took the stand on Monday, February 28, 2000, I told jurors substantially the same thing. "This is not *Quincy*. This is not Jack Klugman playing Quincy," I said, referring to the once-popular TV drama about a coroner who also was a criminalist, a lawyer, a forensic dentist, and a psychiatrist. "In real life, we have all these specialists and we can call on them." On top of that, I testified that I felt it was inappropriate for Dr. Gerber to go to the hospital in the first hours of the murder investigation to question Dr. Sheppard. Once again, I believed that since he wasn't a homicide detective, he shouldn't have been acting like one. I also felt Dr. Gerber's rush to judgment as to who he believed the killer to be was unacceptable. "I would never, and no one in my office would ever express an opinion until someone is arraigned," I said.[13]

During other parts of my testimony, I told jurors how I felt a flashlight could have been the weapon used to fracture Marilyn Sheppard's skull. To help the jury visualize that, I stepped out of the witness box and demonstrated with a 1950s-style flashlight on a model head that had been created to approximate Marilyn Sheppard's head and injuries. Once the first blows fractured her skull, succeeding strikes didn't need to be as powerful to cause more fractures.

During cross-examination, Dever brought up my belief that the killings of John F. Kennedy and Robert Kennedy both were carried out by more than one gunman. I always have been candid about those views and can only assume the prosecutor was trying to somehow undermine my credibility because my beliefs didn't coincide with the "official" versions of those assassinations. But in the end I don't believe he succeeded in getting me to stray from my theories and conclusions in the Sheppard case. That's not to say I went into court with a stubborn attitude and the belief I was there to carry the day for Sam Reese Sheppard. I try to be honest and fair, even when asked a question by opposing counsel that I know may not be helpful to the client for whom I'm working.

Following my testimony, Gilbert called many of the other experts working on the case for Sam Reese Sheppard. Dr. Sobel took the stand the next day and after him came Barton Epstein, a blood spatter expert who was a student of Dr. Kirk's. Epstein conducted tests similar to those his teacher had done forty-five years earlier, regarding blood spatter in the bedroom and the blood trail in the house, and came to some similar conclusions. Epstein also disputed the contention from state witnesses that the bloodstains on Dr. Sheppard's watch were spots made by contact, most likely a bloody finger, as opposed to flying blood.[14]

The trial went on for many more weeks. The attorneys gave closing arguments April 11; the prosecutors stressed Dr. Sheppard's infidelity and dismissed the DNA evidence compiled by Gilbert's team as "mumbo jumbo." Gilbert detailed the many reasons why he said Dr. Sheppard did not kill his wife and reiterated that Dr. Sheppard's blood was not found at the scene.

It didn't seem to matter. The next day, after just three hours of deliberation, the jury returned with its verdict. In a unanimous 8-0 decision, jurors rejected the claim that Dr. Sheppard was innocent of murdering his wife. I wasn't in Cleveland for the verdict, but I spoke with Gilbert soon afterward. Both of us were disappointed, but I can't say I was surprised. The feeling in the community of

Cuyahoga County that Dr. Sheppard killed his wife remains strong even to this day.

Ask folks outside the area whether they believe Dr. Sheppard is innocent and more likely than not, the answer will be yes. But the incredible negative publicity and bias within Cuyahoga County that marked the beginning of this murder investigation seemed unbreakable, despite a ruling by the U.S. Supreme Court and solid forensic evidence.

"One thing an appellate court can't do is change the minds of people," I said. "Once a population has been poisoned, it's been poisoned."

Gilbert agreed with me. He, too, believed that there remains a great deal of latent prejudice in the community and that it found its way into the most recent jury pool. During our conversation and in a letter he wrote to me, Gilbert had a hard time accepting the idea that jurors simply ignored the forensics in the case. But however great his disappointment, Gilbert was left with a sense that all of us working to clear Dr. Sheppard's name still accomplished something meaningful.

"I feel that the work done here will serve as a reminder to future generations of the power of forensic science in getting to the truth—no matter how many years have passed," Gilbert wrote me. "It is my sincere hope that we can continue to work together to promote the cause of using forensic science to exonerate the innocent. For me, the years working on this case have taught me how critical the need to bridge the gap between law and science has become."

I could not agree with him more.

Chapter Five

SHOOT-OUT IN MIRACLE VALLEY

The Killing of Religious Sect Members

WHEN FEDERAL LAW ENFORCEMENT's 1993 INVASION of the Branch Davidian Compound in Waco, Texas, turned tragic, authorities said the event had been totally unpredictable. Never before, they claimed, had they ever had to deal with people so religiously militant and distrusting of government that they would be willing to sacrifice their own lives in a stand for their cause. The U.S. Department of Justice said that the reason it misunderstood and mishandled David Koresh and his followers was simply because it was a unique event in American law enforcement.

However, those claims and excuses were just not true.

A little more than a decade before the confrontation in Waco, and about one thousand miles to the west, an earlier showdown occurred with police. The 1982 confrontation offered a perfect case study for law enforcement on how to react to—and how *not* to react to—religious zealots who feel their faith is being attacked or challenged by Uncle Sam. Federal agents involved in the Branch Davidian siege knew—or at least should have known—about what happened in a small rural town in southern Arizona eleven years before. If they had studied the Arizona case, scores of people probably would not have died in Waco.

But, as is frequently stated, if we do not learn from history, we are doomed to repeat it.

The Arizona situation started almost identically to Waco. A religious sect moves into a small community. Their numbers start to swell among the local population. Confrontations emerge between local residents and the newcomers. Complaints are made to police. Tensions escalate. The newcomers say law enforcement is harassing them because of their faith. Police say that the newcomers think they are above the law.

To show they are in charge, authorities force a showdown. Tempers flare. Weapons are drawn. Shots are fired. People are killed. In this case, ten members of the church faced criminal charges, including allegations of murder. The church had also filed a $75 million civil rights lawsuit against the county.

Lawyers representing the Christ Miracle Healing Center and Church contacted me in the fall of 1983. Armand Salese, a trial attorney from Tucson, Arizona, called me seeking my expert advice and assistance. He told me that my investigation would go directly to the heart of the case. I told Salese I was interested, so he said he would send me some materials in the mail.

On December 1, 1983, I received a package from the Arizona lawyer. Enclosed were statements from the witnesses, the autopsy reports, and twenty-six crime scene photographs. He also included scores of newspaper articles that provided background on the people of Miracle Valley and incidents leading up to the tragic events. The confrontation left two church members dead, each shot multiple times. Another lay dying in a hospital. Two other church members were injured. About ten police officers had also been hurt, though not seriously.

In his letter to me, Salese said he wanted me to review the case and answer eight questions:

1. What was the order of the bullet wounds?
2. What was the track of the bullets through the bodies?
3. Which way did the force of the bullets hitting the bodies turn the bodies?
4. Which of the bullet wounds were fatal?
5. Did certain bullet wounds go from back to front or side to side?
6. How long could the victims have lived after receiving these wounds?
7. Could one of the victims have had a gun in his hand, as claimed by the police officer who shot him?
8. Is it possible that one bullet caused multiple wounds?

"One of the things we need to do is exclude possibilities based upon the pathology of the wounds sustained by the victims," Salese said in the letter.

While it is always the aim of a forensic pathologist to determine what happened in a particular crime or incident, it can be equally important for us to examine the evidence so that we can exclude certain scenarios or claims. Frequently, there is no videotape recording showing what happened without a shadow of a doubt. Nor is there always physical evidence that definitively proves guilt. In many situations, the eyewitness testimony is conflicting. The best the forensic evidence can do is show which side is more likely to be telling the truth.

That was clearly the situation involving the shoot-out in Miracle Valley on October 23, 1982. The charges and countercharges were similar to those in civil rights cases involving police across the country: the police claimed that the church members were a bunch of lawless terrorists carrying guns and other weapons. The officers said that the church members attacked them first and, moreover, that the members of the church were trying to kill them. The sheriff's deputies claimed they shot only in self-defense.

Of course, the church members told a different story. They said it was the police who provoked the confrontation and fired first. They claimed that the three men who were dead did not attack the officers and had not been carrying guns or weapons. Instead, the church argued that the entire confrontation had been preplanned by the sheriff's office to carry out an assassination of church members.

I had first heard about the shooting a few months earlier in the *New York Times*, though the newspaper had published only a few articles about the shoot-out. Yet I was fascinated with the details. The lawyers sent me several boxes of documents and records about the case, including the police reports, sworn statements given by the church members who were present, autopsy reports, and crime scene photographs. In addition, I received scores of articles from the *Arizona Republic*, the state's largest newspaper, and other publications that covered the tragedy.

What I learned certainly intrigued me. I frequently find that a useful way to begin determining what happened in a particular situation, whom to believe and whom to distrust, is to find out as much information as possible about the sources of information. I discovered that the story of what happened in Miracle Valley, Arizona, began long before the explosive showdown in 1982.

In 1958, an old-fashioned tent-revivalist and faith healer named Asa A. Allen moved to Miracle Valley, which is about twenty miles from the Mexico border and about sixty miles southeast of Tucson.

In his autobiography, *Born to Lose, Bound to Win*, Allen claimed that his move from Chicago to Miracle Valley was the result of a miracle directly from heaven. He said that one of his followers who lived in southern Arizona decided to sell his ranch and planned to donate the money to Allen. But at the real estate's closing, the buyer of the property was suddenly struck with blindness. The seller, according to Allen, realized then that he was not supposed to sell the property but that he should donate it to Allen's ministry, A. A. Allen Revivals, Inc. The book also claims that the man who planned to buy the ranch was able to see again only after he agreed not to buy the land.[1]

The ranch consisted of about 1,200 acres of grassland near the foot of the Huachuca Mountains. Allen, whose national television ministry had an annual budget of about $2 million, purchased another 1,200 acres adjacent to the original property. Highway 92 runs right through the heart of the property. The preacher called it "God's home, a beacon for sinners, a refuge for Christians and seekers of the Holy Ghost."[2]

Reverend Allen renamed the roads that zigzagged his property with biblical titles, such as Healing Way, Loaves and Fishes Lane, and Chariot of Fire Drive. Throughout the sixties, the ministry grew, relying heavily on Allen's evangelical and dramatic style. His followers were white and black, wealthy and poor, rural and urban.

In 1970, Allen died, according to the coroner's report, in a hotel room in San Francisco where he was "grossly drunk." He died as the result of damage done by alcoholism. At the time of his death, reports estimated that he had 400,000 followers. His mission had revenues topping $3.5 million. The church employed two hundred and had built a 2,500-seat auditorium. The ministry also built a recording studio and a publishing plant, and it started Southern Arizona Bible College.[3]

Others, including one of Allen's followers, Rev. Don Stewart,

tried to replace their beloved leader. But none had his charisma—or his fundraising capabilities. So the Allen ministries faded. The property in Arizona was auctioned off piece by piece. The college was closed after a fire destroyed much of the campus.

In 1979, Frances Thomas and her son, William, drove their older model tan-and-brown Lincoln Continental from Chicago to Miracle Valley. A short, heavyset, fierce-eyed woman in her fifties (she always refused to give her age, according to news reports), the Reverend Thomas said she "discovered God" and had been healed during one of Allen's revivals.

"We were led by the Lord to come to Arizona because the people would feel freer," William Thomas told the congregation of three hundred who followed them to the Southwest. "We came to fulfill the vision and complete the work of Brother Allen."[4]

They called their new ministry the Christ Miracle and Healing Center Church. They called Miracle Valley "God's City." They remodeled an abandoned restaurant as a church building. They bought a few homes and rented several more. Reverend Thomas, who was the senior pastor, said she preached "nothing but holiness."[5]

The two hundred or so residents of Miracle Valley who did not belong to the church were mostly white and earned low to moderate incomes. They were used to groups moving in and out of their small town, but they had not seen such large numbers of people entering their community since Allen died. Their initial apprehension was replaced by pleasant surprise. Their new neighbors seemed, well, neighborly. The newcomers went to church, attended school board meetings, and seemed to want to become active members of the community.

The church members adopted strict standards. They believed smoking, drinking, and dancing were sins. Cursing was prohibited, rock music was evil, and men and women were required to wear modest clothing. Their children were well behaved and well man-

nered. Many of the newcomers found jobs at nearby factories or in retail shops or restaurants. Local employers told journalists that the church members made good and trusted workers.

As one of the neighbors told reporters, "All I can say is that they're a damn sight better than the hippies that was here before."

But in the spring of 1980, the community suffered from a series of robberies and break-ins—all blamed by local residents on illegal immigrants coming across the nearby border. When the home of church members John and Willie Mae Drew was burglarized, a police report was filed immediately. However, the Cochise County sheriff's office never sent a deputy to investigate, saying its office was seriously underfunded and understaffed.

Citing the increase in crime, leaders of the church met with the sheriff's office to offer to patrol the streets at night as a private security force. The sheriff's office quickly accepted the offer, thinking the patrols would be similar to other neighborhood crime watch programs. At first, most local residents praised the church members for being so community-minded and thanked them for the neighborhood patrols.

However, there were some local residents who were upset by the newcomers from day one. Bear in mind, the church's presence suddenly changed the racial makeup of the previously all-white Miracle Valley. By the winter of 1980, tension had gripped the tiny town. There had been a handful of minor confrontations between white residents and black church members—most of them nonviolent. The number of security patrols increased. Local residents complained that the church members participating in the twenty-four-hour patrols were taking advantage of Arizona's liberal gun laws by dangerously arming themselves.

Residents complained to authorities that the church security patrols were conducting frequent roadblocks. They were stopping and searching cars. If they didn't recognize the passengers, the armed patrols would escort the vehicles to the city limits. Newspaper deliverers, water company workers, and United Parcel Service drivers reported that they were constantly being harassed by the patrols.

As more and more church members moved to Miracle Valley, the residents felt the church was using the patrols to intimidate them. The longtimers felt the church members were trying to force them to leave the town so that the church would be able to purchase their property at bargain prices. The problem, according to the police and local residents, was that church members wanted to create their own law and that they didn't care if they ran over the local residents.

For their part, church members complained that there was a conspiracy among county officials to force them out of Miracle Valley. Church leaders felt they were being discriminated against, either because of their religious beliefs or because of the color of their skin or both. They filed a $75 million civil rights lawsuit against the county, accusing county leaders of restructuring zoning ordinances to severely restrict mobile homes in Miracle Valley. Since mobile homes were the preferred residence of most church members because it was all they could afford, the county was, in essence, using the law to limit the number of church members who could live in Miracle Valley.

The church's lawsuit also charged the sheriff's office with violating the civil rights and civil liberties of its members. The complaint accused Cochise County sheriff Jimmy Judd of targeting church members in enforcing traffic codes and other Arizona criminal laws.

Sheriff Judd was the epitome of the Western lawman. He was never seen without his cowboy hat. His bulldog face and homespun manner made him a political favorite. The church members said the sheriff's office was nothing more than a "good ole boy" system filled with racist officers. In 1975, Cochise County had adopted an affirmative action program. However, the program had included only women and Latinos, not black people.[6]

The real escalation in tension occurred in the spring of 1981. The Arizona Department of Economic Security Administration investigated the deaths of five children from the church over a period of several months. The inquiry focused on the death of six-year-old Theriel Drew. The boy suffered from a strangulated hernia. Church members didn't believe in medical care or medicines as treatment.

For four days, neighbors said they heard the young boy screaming from intense and agonizing pain. Authorities determined that the deaths of Theriel and the four others were needless, because their sicknesses could have been treated with medicine and their deaths could have been easily prevented.

Church members said they believed in faith healing only. If they treated their illnesses with conventional medicine, the members believed they were directly violating biblical commandments. It was God's will, they told police, for the children to die. And they pointed to other children who had also been extremely sick, but faith healing had cured them.[7]

The state officials didn't accept the answer. The authorities filed documents in court saying they needed to take custody of a select number of other children in order to protect them from the alleged neglect. When church members ignored the court orders, sheriff's deputies drove to Miracle Valley to remove the children from their homes. But as the officers approached the houses, they were quickly surrounded by church members carrying baseball bats. They would not allow their children to be taken. They vowed to die before they would allow the children to go, and they threatened to kill the deputies if the officers tried to take the children by force.

At a county school board meeting a few weeks later at the Palemino School, tempers flared inside and outside the building.

Inside, church members tried to explain to other residents their beliefs about faith healing. But many of the residents quickly dismissed the church's view and referred to them as a "cult."

Outside the school in the parking lot, a Cochise County sheriff's deputy claimed that George Smith, a member of the church who had been inside at the school board meeting, threw gravel at him by spinning his car wheels as he left the parking lot. The deputy also said he saw Smith driving through a stop sign without stopping. However, two officers with the Arizona Department of Public Safety testified in court that the car didn't throw gravel at all, nor did they see Smith run a stop sign.[8]

Even so, the deputy jumped in his patrol car and chased Smith into Miracle Valley, with his lights flashing and siren blaring. The deputy reported that he pulled Smith over but that Smith refused to get out of the car. When he tried to pull Smith out of the car by force, he was attacked by two women from the church who were walking nearby. He reported that the women punched him in the face and tried to stab him with a pair of scissors; then his nightstick was taken away and he was surrounded and threatened by thirty black church members. He immediately jumped in his car and retreated.

The next day, August 25, 1981, Sheriff Judd called public safety officials to request that additional state officers be assigned to the area to help him patrol Miracle Valley. When a handful of state police officers arrived, they discovered the sheriff's SWAT team was carrying loaded machine guns and high-powered rifles; they were hiding in the bushes and weeds in Miracle Valley to monitor church members. Other witnesses said armed deputies would frequently stand on the roof of the nearby Palomino School or on a nearby tower, using binoculars and rifles with high-powered scopes to watch church members in Miracle Valley.

It was about this time that Cochise County authorities started posting new traffic signs in Miracle Valley that intensified the bad feelings of church members, according to the federal lawsuit filed by the church. The traffic postings were simply "pedestrian crossing" signs. But the depiction on the signs could be taken as nothing less than racially demeaning and offensive to people of color.

The signs, which were posted only in Miracle Valley but no other part of all-white Cochise County, depicted two adults and two children crossing a street. The sign had the words "Slow Down: Children Playing." But the three people depicted on the sign were black with large white eyes and mouths. The children were wearing T-shirts with the letter "N" on them. Church members complained that the people on the signs looked like Al Jolson and that the "N" on the clothes stood for "nigger."[9]

On August 27, George Smith peacefully turned himself in to the police. He paid the traffic fine without any confrontations, arguments, or griping. Tensions were mounting in the valley. People were openly talking about an armed showdown between the church members and either the police or the local residents.

There's no question that the members of the church developed a more militant attitude. William Thomas Jr., son of the church leader, a father of five, and one of the assistant pastors in the church, wrote the following letter to the congregation:

> We are a humble people, bringing the things we could carry. Peace and harmony we offered. They came into our church and we welcomed them. Then beneath their smiling faces came the anger hidden deep. They watched our homes, harassed our children, and followed behind us in the street. Should we stay and give a fight or give up what's our own? Should we stand up and be recognized or bend beneath the white's bar?

The letter, which was later introduced as evidence in court, became a rallying point for church members, who started training in the martial arts. The church adopted a "Commando Code" for its members to learn and recite: "I am a commando for Christ. I serve in the holiness which guards the saints and God's Valley and God's way of life. If I am captured, I will resist by every means available, I am willing to give my life."[10]

But the church and its members were not without blame. On several occasions, church members surrounded the cars of police officers simply trying to do their duties, including officers who were sympathetic to the causes of the church. The officers said they felt that the church members were trying to intimidate them and prevent them from enforcing state laws.

The church suffered tremendously when a television crew that had been reporting the tensions in Miracle Valley stopped along Highway 92, which runs through the center of the community. While video-taping the landscape, the photographer was attacked by five female church members who hit him with hammers and clubs. The entire event was captured on video and replayed over and over on the local television news. It was clear on the tape that the photographer did not instigate the confrontation, nor did he do anything to anger the women.

The next Sunday morning, Rev. Frances Thomas preached that "these niggers are not going to run. Reporters try to make us look like criminals," according to court records. Clearly, neither the church nor the local authorities were willing to accept responsibility for their shortcomings or wrongdoings.

In September 1981 a series of events rippled through the church and local community that would lay the basis for the tragic events that would occur a year later. It started the night of September 7, when police received calls that shots had been fired from a vehicle cruising the Valley. Deputies and state patrol officers, including state officer Thad Hall, raced into the Valley. The church's armed force moved quickly to seal off all roads going in and out of the Valley. No one was allowed to leave.

Just as the officers arrived, the church's security force stopped a pickup truck. The passenger, a drunken white woman, started using racially offensive language toward the church's security guards. One of the black security guards, obviously offended and aggravated, told the white woman she should step outside the vehicle. That's when Officer Hall immediately intervened. He told the church member to back away, that he would take care of it. Hall later testified that the church member obeyed, and that was the extent of the confrontation. The vehicle was searched but no gun was found.

Three days later, a deputy with the Cochise County sheriff's office filed charges against Sherman McCane, a member of the church's security force who had stopped the vehicle. The deputy, in a written report, said McCane assaulted him while the vehicle was being searched. "I felt my life was in danger," the deputy wrote.

McCane and his wife, Susie, were arrested on September 10 and charged with assaulting a police officer. But the charge against Susie McCane, which was later disclosed to be perjury, seemed incredibly bizarre. The facts of this incident indicated to me that the officials in Cochise County were so opposed or biased against the members of the Christ Miracle Church that they were willing to do whatever it took to punish the members and run them out of town.[11]

The perjury charge stemmed from the fact that the McCanes were allowing a relative's four children to live with them. The children's mother had died and the father was living somewhere in Mississippi, trying to get his life together. When Susie tried to get the children admitted to the Cochise public schools, she was told they would not be allowed to attend because their legal guardian was not living in Arizona.

To correct the situation, Susie visited a lawyer to obtain temporary guardianship so that the children would be admitted to school. The appropriate documents were filed. That's when prosecutors and police got involved. They claimed that Susie lied in the documents about not knowing the address of the children's father. The authorities claimed that Susie knew the father lived in Mississippi.

The charges against Susie were eventually dismissed after her lawyer stepped forward criticizing the local authorities, according to court records. The lawyer said the error was his doing, not the fault of Susie McCane. He said that when he filled out the paperwork, he asked Susie if she knew the address of the children's father. Susie told the lawyer she thought he lived in Mississippi but that she didn't know his exact address. The lawyer says he wrote "address unknown" on the filing. In essence, the lawyer testified that Cochise County officials were prosecuting Susie McCane for trying to help four children get an education.

But before the McCane's case could be worked out, authorities took away the four children, placing them in police custody. The children were kept at a hotel in nearby Sierra Vista. The kids later testified that the police officers offered them candy and other treats if they would say on tape that they had seen their parents and other church members carrying guns and making threats. On tape, the children steadfastly denied they had witnessed such things.

The next day, a group of church members gathered in Miracle Valley. They were convinced that the charges against the McCanes were fabricated and frivolous. They further believed their fellow church members were the targets of selective prosecution and would be railroaded through the criminal justice system.

On September 11 several church members packed into a van and headed toward Sierra Vista, where the McCanes were being held in jail. Just a few miles down the road, a bomb exploded inside the van. Several church members were injured. Steve Lindsay, a twenty-one-year-old member of the church, died instantly, according to the medical examiner's report, when the bomb literally blew him apart. Authorities contended that the bomb, which consisted of several sticks of dynamite, was in his lap when it detonated.

Sheriff's deputies and some local residents immediately specu-
lated that the church members were on their way to the jail to free
the McCanes. Church leaders adamantly denied it. In fact, Reverend Thomas said the bomb had been planted in the van by others.

McCane was found guilty a few weeks later. It certainly seemed
as if the church's fears of police intimidation and discrimination
were proven true in this case. I learned that Officer Hall of the state
police had filed a report with the local prosecutor informing her that
he was with McCane and the deputy who claimed he was assaulted
on September 7.

In his report, Officer Hall said he never saw McCane and the
deputy involved in a confrontation. Despite this obviously relevant
evidence, the prosecutor did not call Officer Hall to testify at the
trial, nor did she inform lawyers for McCane about Officer Hall's
statement.

Tensions seemed to ease throughout the winter, however. To
help facilitate better communications, Arizona governor Bruce
Babbitt sent a trained mediator, who also happened to be a black
police officer, to Miracle Valley to meet with both sides. For three
days, the mediator got Sheriff Judd and Reverend Thomas to air
their grievances in a private conference room at a local motel.

The negotiations ended with both sides holding a joint press
conference announcing they had worked out an agreement. Both
sides said they were making concessions. Under the "Memorandum
of Understanding," Sheriff Judd promised to hire black deputies
who would be trained to handle the special needs of their community. The sheriff also agreed to open a precinct in Miracle Valley.
Thomas said she agreed that the church would disband its security
patrols and would open a better dialogue with local authorities and
residents.

But the agreement wasn't worth the paper it was printed on.
Neither side took a single step toward implementing the deal. No

black officers were hired, and the church never stopped its armed patrols.

Over the next several months, state officials tried again and again to act as mediators between the church members and the sheriff's office, but Sheriff Judd was under intense pressure from local white citizens to crack down on the church members. The state police officers, many of whom were black, said the local deputies were filled with hatred and racist views toward the church members. Officer Hall heard one deputy ask, "How are the natives doing up there?"

Sgt. Bill Fogel, who headed the regional office of the Arizona Department of Public Safety, said Sheriff Judd "asked the Governor for a tank to go into the Valley to annihilate those niggers. That is exactly what he said." Each time, Governor Babbitt turned him down.[12]

Meanwhile, the Christ Miracle Church was going through an internal power struggle. While Rev. Frances Thomas was advocating less confrontation, her son, William Thomas Jr., favored a much more militant style. In a written sermon delivered in September 1982, the younger Thomas seemed to predict his own death.

"I find that death sings a sweeter song and plays a softer tone than the cold iron chains of slavery," he said. "We are branded a cult because they say we are chanting and we are said to be lunatics. I find they have conspired to re-oppress and enslave us like they have the Mexicans and Indians. I find Hitler is very much alive and well in Cochise County. And I say it is you Hitler, who disguises himself as our county official, it is you who judges us today but it is God who will judge you tomorrow."

Sheriff Judd, feeling he was losing support among white voters, realized he needed to do something. He decided it was time to take action. The sun was setting on southern Arizona on October 22 when Sheriff Judd sent two of his deputies to Miracle Valley to arrest church member Frank Bernard on a traffic warrant. The specific charge: driving with a suspended license.

As two deputies pulled up to Bernard's home, their patrol car was quickly surrounded by a handful of black men and women. The deputies warned the church members to stand back. The congregation ignored the officers' instructions. The deputies radioed back to the station that they were under attack. Sheriff Judd ordered his officers to withdraw.

That night, the sheriff called an editor at the *Arizona Daily Star* asking him to hold off publishing an article about the incident. Judd told the newspaper that his office was making plans to raid the church's compound the next day. But the editor, worried that there might be trouble brewing in Miracle Valley, called the governor's office.

Governor Babbitt called Judd directly. "Let's talk about this," the governor told the sheriff. "There's no reason to do anything rash."

"I've had enough talk," Judd responded. "I'm going to show the people of Miracle Valley that I'm the law."

Governor Babbitt, who later ran for president and who became the interior secretary under President Clinton, didn't get much sleep that night. He stayed on the telephone all night trying to spark interest in negotiations.

Late that night, Sheriff Judd called all his deputies to come to the office. Many of his deputies lived in Bisbee, while others resided in Sierra Vista. Miracle Valley is between the two.

"For over two years, law enforcement and the local community of Miracle Valley and the citizens of the state of Arizona have bent over backwards to say welcome to the Miracle Valley newcomers," the sheriff told a reporter that night. "During this time, citizens have not freely walked their home streets. Needless deaths have occurred on several occasions. The public at large has been placed in grave danger by the lawless activities of church members."

The next morning, Saturday, October 23, Cochise County deputies moved into place about 9 A.M. All roads leaving Miracle Valley were sealed off, and Miracle Valley was surrounded. Deputy Pat Halloran and Capt. Bert Goodman slowly drove into Miracle Valley to arrest Bernard on a traffic violation. But Bernard wasn't there.

Instead, one hundred church members surrounded them. The officers called for backup. Deputies immediately flooded the valley, but the church members seemed prepared for the onslaught. The mediator from the governor's office had called church leaders to warn them.

All hell broke loose. About fifty deputies raided the church's campus. They were fully armed with riot helmets, bulletproof vests, M-16s, AR-15s, an Uzi, and M-14s. The church members had rocks, sticks, baseball bats, clubs, and at least two guns. Melee erupted. There was shouting. People were taking swings at each other. And then it happened: bullets suddenly filled the air.

As more church members rushed out of their homes and toward the deputies, Sheriff Judd called for an immediate retreat. They took with them nine church members, who were placed under arrest for assault.

The sheriff initially announced that twenty-five of his deputies had been injured. That number was later reduced to seven. Two had gunshot wounds, five suffered broken bones, and only one deputy had to be hospitalized. By contrast, two church members lay in the high grass field, dead from bullets. Two other church members were injured, though not seriously, and a third man was in critical condition, a bullet in his spine. He would later die.

What happened that day in Miracle Valley depends upon whom you ask.

The first eyewitness account made public was that of *Arizona Daily Star* reporter Paul Brinkley-Rogers, who accompanied deputies into the Valley to see what would happen. His front-page account in the next morning's newspaper was chilling.

"The shooting started with the pop of a gunshot to the rear of the quiet residential neighborhood," Brinkley-Rogers wrote. "Then another pop from somewhere else. The officers, fighting with the yelling, kicking, screaming, spitting mob of men, women, and children, tried to push them away and level their weapons at the sounds of the shots at the same time."

The journalist told about an older female church member he had met and talked to several times coming toward him in a threatening manner. "You are writing your last story, Paul," he quoted her as yelling. "You're hell-bound. You'll pay for this, just like the others, and I will send you to hell. If I don't kill you today, I'll kill you tomorrow."

Brinkley-Rogers also described an "angry woman waving a rake at a young deputy like a spear. The woman lunged at him, calling him a 'filthy honky killer.' The deputy used the butt of his Mini-14, a semi-automatic rifle, to crack her on the jaw and knock her to the ground. Then he turned toward the popping shots and pulled his trigger."

"The woman on the ground grabbed his ankles and pulled the deputy to the ground. Another woman with a rock banged away at the deputy's gold-colored crash helmet. Children jumped on his back and tore at his clothes." He wrote that "each deputy was fighting off three or four attackers.

"There were bursts of rifle fire. A Mini-14 firing on the right. A 30-caliber carbine pumping away. People staggered and ran for cover. They looked at one another to see if they had been shot. Men and women were wailing. Finally, the deputies were ready to pull out.

"Let's make sure we haven't left anybody in the grass," he quoted a deputy as yelling in retreat.

Reverend Thomas told a different account about what happened to the *Chicago Sun-Times*. "The deputies came in and just started shooting people down like dogs," she said. "A policeman started shooting everybody. One cop, he had a machine gun, was shooting. Another cop yelled, 'Don't shoot these people.'"

Once the law enforcement officers had fled the area, the church members searched their wounded. They found thirty-three-year-old William Thomas Jr., the son of the founder, lying dead. So was Aguster Tate, a fifty-two-year-old follower. Another church member, Roy Williams, was barely moving. Two other church members were bleeding.

State police immediately flooded the Valley. Local residents were evacuated, and church members were told to remain in their homes. Governor Babbitt asked the FBI to investigate what had happened. By nightfall, total quiet had descended on Miracle Valley.

The NAACP called the shootings a "premeditated police-state action." Jesse Jackson said, "It was clear to us that people were being driven from their homes. They lived there in fear and apprehension. They were shot in the back. This is one of the greatest tragedies of our time."[13]

Cochise County prosecutors sought and got indictments against ten church members. The charges included assault on police officers and attempted murder. At the same time, federal agents opened an inquiry about whether the sheriff and his deputies had violated federal civil rights laws. And lawyers for the church amended their $75 million lawsuit to include the police raid and the three deaths.

It was in regard to those three cases that I was contacted by Armand Salese, the Tucson lawyer representing the church for free. He was defending the church members against the criminal charges, as well as pursuing the civil claims on behalf of church members.

My role was to examine competing statements made by Cochise County deputy Ray Thatcher and a handful of church members. Thatcher had fired the bullets that struck and killed William Thomas Jr. and Aguster Tate.

Deputy Thatcher gave a thirty-seven-page statement four days after the shoot-out occurred. His job that day, he said, was to back up the officers who went in to serve the warrant. He went to the scene only after the first two deputies called for help.

"Immediately, black women, I would say ten of them, and one black man, came running up and said for us to get out of their yard," Thatcher said in his statement. "They all had rocks in their hands. I stepped out of the vehicle with my rifle in my hand. I was to cover people and help them get out of the Valley. The women began pelting us with rocks. How many hit me, I have no idea. I guess ten or fifteen rocks at least. Big rocks."

It was then that Deputy Thatcher said he saw a black male toting a rifle coming toward him. "I wanted to get away from that man," he continued. "But he turned and came toward me and he lifted the rifle up and at that time, my rifle came up from the hip where I kept it. I just raised it slightly. And I fired at the man. I think three shots, but I'm not sure. He fell backwards and he fell down. He tried to push himself off the ground. And he had the Winchester rifle raised up off the ground and I shot him again."

"At that time, another black man came running toward me, and ran by me and ran over and knelt down to pick up the Winchester or lever action rifle that was still cocked," Thatcher said in the report. "He grabbed the rifle up from the ground from next to the fellow I had shot and turned toward me, kind of from a kneeling position. He was just in a crouch and turned toward me and raised the rifle. Again, I just turned my rifle slightly to the left and again I fired. And he dropped."

Later in his statement, Deputy Thatcher repeated that both men were facing him when he shot them. "I recall seeing the rounds hit him in the center of the chest," he stated. "I saw the shirt pucker out."

By contrast, four church members who witnessed the shooting had given sworn statements that William Thomas, the church's co-pastor, was facing away from Deputy Thatcher throughout the entire episode. The witnesses said that Thomas was waving church members to get back and that he had nothing in his hands, including no gun, as Thatcher claimed. The witnesses also claimed that Aguster Tate never threatened Deputy Thatcher. Instead, he rushed to help the injured Thomas, who was also Tate's son-in-law. Tate was facing away from Thatcher, the witnesses stated, when Thatcher fired on him.

Salese also included a photograph that was published on the front page of the *Arizona Republic* the night of the melee. The picture shows the pandemonium of the event. But after a closer look, I quickly understood why lawyers found the photograph so fascinating. In it, William Thomas is shown waving his arms toward church members telling them to retreat to their homes. The picture supported the church members' statements.

As I reviewed the statements, I noticed two additional documents. The first was documentation that the church members had passed a polygraph test with flying colors. It is true that polygraph tests are seldom admissible in court as evidence; however, law enforcement officials rely on them quite often in eliminating suspects.

Lawyers for the church hired the certified polygraphist about five weeks after the incident to question three key eyewitnesses to the shooting.

Question 1: "Did William Thomas Jr. have a weapon in his hand when he was shot?"

Answer: "No."

Question 2: "Was William Thomas Jr. shot in the back by the police officer?"

Answer: "Yes."

Question 3: "Did you see the police officer shoot William Thomas Jr.?"

Answer: "Yes."

Question 4: "Did William Thomas Jr. have his back to the police officer when he was shot?"

Answer: "Yes."

The polygraphist wrote that, in her opinion, the witnesses answered "all of the questions truthfully."

The second document included statements from a Cochise County sheriff's deputy named Matthew Perry. Deputy Perry signed a sworn statement that Thatcher had told him six months earlier that he would kill Thomas if he had the chance.

"We were sitting in his car and he had a rifle," Perry stated. "He reached over and patted the rifle and made statements to the effect that 'those people have ruined this Valley. Those bastards have to go. When the shooting starts, I'm going to get Thomas Junior. I'm going to kill the bastard; he's mine.'"

Pretty damning evidence, to be sure.

I found the most convincing evidence in the science. The autopsy report, completed by Dr. Richard Friede, included photographs of the deceased, x-rays, and the Arizona medical examiner's findings.

William Thomas was shot four times. The first bullet severed the top of his right index finger. The second bullet hit him just above the wrist on his right arm. Bullet three entered his left lower back and went forward through his left kidney. The final bullet also hit him in the back just below the right shoulder.

Tate suffered three bullet wounds. The first entered his upper right torso, just below the base of the neck. The second and third wounds entered the body on the side and traveled sideways. Not one of the bullets traveled from front to back.

On December 12, 1983, I flew to Phoenix to meet with prosecutors and lawyers involved in the Miracle Valley case. For more than two hours, I answered their questions under oath. Salese wanted prosecutors to meet with me prior to trial, in part, to let them know I would be testifying as an expert in the upcoming trial. But Salese was also hoping that the prosecutor would hear my testimony and be convinced to drop the charges against his clients. This kind of pretrial deposition in a criminal case is highly unusual.

The first several minutes were spent establishing my credentials as a forensic pathologist. I walked the lawyers through my educational history and training, followed by various career experiences and professional acknowledgments. In order to be recognized as a medical expert qualified to give opinions, I had to establish my qualifications.

"Is there anything in Dr. Friede's autopsy reports that you disagree with?" Arizona assistant state attorney general Stan Patchell asked.

"No," I responded. "I'm accepting of his descriptions and findings, and I can't think of a single thing that I disagree with. The autopsy was thorough and very professionally completed."

In many cases, experts are called to testify in an effort to undermine the credibility of the prosecution's forensic pathologist or to criticize how the autopsy was performed. I've done that several times in cases where I thought the medical examiner was incompetent or where I believed the autopsy was shabbily done. But this was not one of those situations. Dr. Friede was well respected and the autopsy and medical investigation were expertly conducted.

"Have you concluded, based on all of the evidence you have looked at, whether Mr. Thomas or Mr. Tate was shot first?" the prosecutor inquired.

"I cannot be absolutely certain from a forensic pathology standpoint alone," I answered. "Taking the autopsy reports by themselves, I can't tell you who was shot first."

"Is there anything that you know of, from your examination of all the materials, that would exclude Detective Thatcher's statement that Mr. Thomas was the first person shot?"

"My answer is no," I responded. "There is nothing in those materials or discussions that would cause me to doubt that Thomas was shot first."

The truth was that there was no dispute over who was shot first. Prosecutors and sheriff's deputies tried to say that the evidence supported Thatcher's claim that he shot Thomas first and Tate second. The forensic evidence neither supported nor contradicted this scenario. But it didn't matter because the church members also testified that Thomas was shot first, followed by Tate.

Similarly, the order in which the gunshot wounds were inflicted was inconsequential. There was nothing in the forensic evidence that indicated which wound came first, second, third, or fourth for either Thomas or Tate. Any of them could have been the first bullet without altering the scenario proposed by the church members. By contrast, none of the bullet wounds coming first would have supported Thatcher's account. As a matter of scientific evidence, the sequence of the bullet wounds could not have altered Thomas's or Tate's positioning when they were shot.

Which led, of course, to the most important question: What were the two victims doing when they were shot?

"Now, Dr. Wecht, Detective Thatcher gave a version of the shootings which I think you are aware of," Patchell continued. "He said in both shootings that the men he shot had a gun and were pointing the gun at him. Do you find anything from your examination that would be inconsistent with that?"

"Yes, many things," I answered. "There are things about Thatcher's version or account of the shooting that I do not accept. It's quite clear to me that two of the four wounds could not have been sustained by Thomas under any conceivable circumstances had he been facing Thatcher.

"Thatcher also talks about Thomas having a gun, facing him, with the gun upraised and pointing at Thatcher," I continued. "The problem is the wound Thomas suffered on his right wrist. There is no way that I can think of with Thomas having held a gun and facing Thatcher, that a bullet could have entered into the right wrist and emerged at a lower point than the point that it entered. It just doesn't fit."

For several minutes, I gave the lawyers a quick lesson in anatomy and the trajectory that bullets take. I gave similar testimony regarding the wounds suffered by Aguster Tate. I told them that the first bullet entered his back near the base of his neck and traveled forward. It would have been impossible for the bullet to have taken this course if Tate had been facing Thatcher, as the deputy said.

Prosecutors also questioned me about Detective Thatcher's claim that the two victims pointed guns at him and that he was holding his rifle from the waist when he fired on them.

"I'm familiar with the way that people stand when they are shooting guns," Patchell said. "That is, sideways. They stand sideways to the object they're shooting at."

"Yes, I realize that some people turn more sideways when they fire a gun," I responded. "But that isn't Thatcher's description about what happened."

At the request of prosecutors, I then spent several minutes tracking each bullet through the bodies of Thomas and Tate. The bullets generally moved from back to front, right to left. While all four bullet wounds contradicted Thatcher's scenario regarding what happened, "wound C," as labeled by Dr. Friede, provided the clearest evidence.

"[The bullet that caused] wound C entered the right side of the back approximately twenty inches from the top of the head and six inches to the right of the mid vertebral line," I told prosecutors. "After entering the right side of the back it went on an angle from right to left and at a slightly downward track. It went through the skin, through fat and muscle, passed just below the tenth rib on the right side. The rib was fractured but not shattered, indicating that the bullet probably didn't go through it.

"The bullet then went through the middle and lower lobes of the right lung, and finally fragmented in the left lobe of the liver. If the bullet had stayed together and exited the body, it would have exited somewhere just below the left nipple."

Similarly, I tracked "bullet D," which entered the lower left back about four inches from the side. The bullet went through the skin, fat, and muscle. It then hit the vertebrae at about the belt line. The bony arches at the root of the spinal canal had been shattered. Once again, this proved that Thomas was facing away from Thatcher when he was shot.

Then prosecutors turned their attention to the three wounds suffered by Aguster Tate. I walked the lawyers through each wound. Gunshot wound one entered just below the left shoulder and moved through the armpit, causing significant damage to the lung and the aorta, before finally coming to rest in the right chest. Bullet wound two grazed Tate's right bicep and hand. While neither of these wounds supported Thatcher's account of the shooting, Tate's third bullet wound presented clear and convincing evidence that Tate also had his back to the detective.

"[The bullet that caused] wound three entered the right back about eleven inches below the top of the head and about one inch to the right of the mid-line," I testified under oath. "The bullet traveled through the soft fatty tissue and was recovered in the front chest. So, there's no way that you can have him facing Thatcher or with his side to him or anything like that. The only way for this wound to be inflicted is for Tate to have his back to the officer."

"So your testimony is that there is no evidence that supports Detective Thatcher's statement about what happened?" Patchell inquired. "So, your statement is that Detective Thatcher's statement is a complete lie, that none of it is true?"

"I'm not coming to court to express any psychological opinions about who is and who is not a liar," I concluded. "But my view is that the forensic evidence as I see it scientifically repudiates Thatcher's accounts. I would state with reasonable medical certainty that the Thatcher version is completely inconsistent with any of these shots being fired as the first shots."

"Is there anything you think the church members and Detective Thatcher agree on?" the prosecutor asked.

"About the only thing that they agree on is they were all there and there was a shooting," I responded, partially joking.

That concluded the lengthy sworn deposition. Prosecutors said they would review my testimony in considering whether to continue with the case. If the matter did go to trial, they said I definitely would be called as a witness.

But it never came to that. Just weeks later, state prosecutors dismissed the charges against the ten church members. It was clear to everyone that local law enforcement had not been truthful about what happened on October 23, 1982, in Miracle Valley.

That important decision was followed weeks later by another. County officials decided to settle the church's lawsuit. The terms of the deal were never disclosed, though I would bet they were favorable to church members. The decision by the county to settle was encouraged by the federal judge who ruled that he believed that Sheriff Judd's office was permeated with racism. The judge concluded his case with one final sentence:

"It seems to me that everyone in Cochise County decided they were going to get in their licks against the church one way or another."[14]

Chapter Six

STANDING BY HER MAN

Tammy Wynette's Final Song

I F THE LIFE OF COUNTRY MUSIC LEGEND Tammy Wynette were ever reduced to lyrics and put to music, it likely would be a hit on the country charts. It contains all the elements: a humble beginning; success; troubles with men, money, and painkillers; and, finally, a sad ending. But Wynette's life was no honky-tonk tune. And some of the questions raised after her death at age fifty-five were more suited to a John Grisham novel than a song.

In the immediate aftermath of Wynette's passing on April 6, 1998, at her home in Nashville, there was only sorrow. Fans and fellow performers mourned the woman known as the "first lady of country music" through tributes and memorial services. Stories that ran in newspapers across the nation noted Wynette's improbable rise from a child living on a cotton farm in Mississippi to a beautician in Birmingham, Alabama, to a beloved singer who recorded more than fifty albums and sold more than thirty million records.

The articles also noted Wynette had suffered from chronic health problems and that she probably died from a blood clot while sleeping. The singer of such classics as "Stand by Your Man" and "D-I-V-O-R-C-E" was embalmed and laid to rest within days. No autopsy was conducted.

In the world of country music, everyone knew Tammy Wynette. At a memorial service, Dolly Parton remembered recording the album "Honky Tonk Angels" with Wynette and Loretta Lynn. "Tammy was like family to me. She was like a little sister and I loved her dearly," Parton said, her voice filled with emotion. "We had a lot of laughs together. We were just silly girls."

Randy Travis, another country music singer and friend, also spoke. "Tammy was a wonderful lady and a lot of people who didn't know her, who didn't get to spend the time around her that I did . . . didn't get to see the sense of humor," he said. "She was a lady who enjoyed laughing, as well as [her husband] George, and we all did have a lot of good laughs together."

Before the laughs, however, there was hard work. She was born Virginia Wynette Pugh and spent her early years picking cotton on her family's farm in Itawamba County, Mississippi. She married just before graduating high school and soon had two daughters. By 1965, she had three daughters and was divorced. The next year, she moved to Nashville to pursue her dreams of being a singer. Wynette auditioned for famed producer Billy Sherrill, and that same year, 1966, she released her first single, "Apartment #9." After that, there was no turning back.

Wynette's career immediately took off. She recorded albums that became number-one hits, and in 1968 started a relationship with her idol, country singer George Jones. They soon married, her third marriage, but it was a relationship with many ups and downs, and they divorced in 1975. After a brief fourth marriage, Wynette wed George Richey in 1978. Richey had been friends with Wynette for many years, and he and his prior wife socialized with Wynette and Jones. Richey also was in the entertainment business, a successful songwriter and producer who once served as musical director of the TV show *Hee Haw*.

But Wynette's personal tribulations did not impede her professional achievements. During her career, she collected two Grammy awards and numerous Country Music Association awards, and performed for five presidents, from Gerald Ford to Bill Clinton. She also acted, performing on the CBS soap opera *Capitol* in the 1980s and appearing on the sitcom *Evening Shade*.

All the while, Wynette battled health problems. After the birth of her fourth daughter in 1970, she had an appendectomy and hysterectomy, surgeries that never healed properly. During a twenty-five-year period, Wynette underwent more than thirty operations to try to correct health problems and alleviate the pain, but they didn't really help enough.[1] She turned to prescription pain pills, which led to a stay in the Betty Ford Clinic in the 1980s.

In the nineties, Wynette made a brief departure from her country roots to record a duet with an English pop group called KLF. The song, "Justified & Ancient," became a number-one hit in eighteen countries. But the new decade also brought more medical complications, this time bile duct infections. At the end of 1993, Wynette was admitted to a hospital in Nashville and nearly died. After several days, during which her condition was too precarious to operate, doctors finally were able to take her into surgery and remove some of the scar tissue in her abdomen that was causing a blockage.

So even though Wynette had a long and complicated medical history, after she died, three of her four daughters began asking questions about the circumstances surrounding her death. They knew she had medical problems, but none of them believed those difficulties were life threatening. In fact, Wynette reportedly had been feeling better and performing in the months prior to her death.

The daughters—Jackie Daly, Tina Jones, and Georgette Smith—also knew their mother was on many medications to control her pain. But they wanted to find out just how much she had been given and why several of the more powerful narcotics were never listed on an initial police report taken the night of her death.

They further questioned why Wynette's personal physician, Dr. Wallis Marsh, flew 470 miles from Pittsburgh that spring night to pronounce her dead and sign the death certificate. Marsh, who had been treating Wynette since 1992, concluded without an internal exam that she died of a pulmonary embolism—a blood clot.

Her daughters believed an autopsy would go a long way toward answering their questions, but there were obstacles. George Richey opposed exhuming her body. Medical examiner Dr. Bruce Levy accepted that Wynette died of natural causes and was not inclined to pursue having her disinterred. The women turned to the media, and the media turned to me.

In early 1999, producers for the ABC news program *20/20* contacted me and asked if I would be willing to review some of the facts in the Tammy Wynette case and to offer my opinions. I frequently receive calls from newspaper, radio, and television reporters seeking a comment about a case in their area or one that has garnered national attention. If possible, I try to accommodate them. Sometimes news agencies even send me materials and ask for an opinion on a particular situation.

Such was the circumstance in 1991 when the *San Francisco Examiner* approached me. The newspaper at the time had just won a fight to gain access to the autopsy reports of forty-two people who died when a viaduct collapsed on dozens of cars during the 1989 Loma Prieta earthquake. The paper's reporters were investigating how well prepared emergency rescue officials were to deal with such a natural disaster. They wanted me to review those autopsy reports to see how long any of the victims could have survived after the collapse. It was a significant amount of work and I wasn't paid, but I agreed to do it because I felt it could provide some public-safety benefit.

What I found troubled me. After reviewing all forty-two cases, I believed that as many as nine of the victims could have survived their injuries if rescue crews had done their jobs quickly and efficiently, and gotten to them in the rubble. Many of the victims lived for hours after the quake and probably suffered great pain before expiring.

The Tammy Wynette case was not quite the same type of case, but I nonetheless agreed to look over the police reports and her death certificate. Several aspects of the case aroused my suspicions. For one, I had never heard of a doctor getting on a plane and flying somewhere to declare a person dead. Second, I had a problem with Dr. Marsh opining that Wynette died of a pulmonary embolism without having performed an autopsy.

"It's no more than an educated guess," I told the *20/20* camera crew for the show that aired February 19, 1999.

"So it would be impossible to diagnose by just looking at Tammy Wynette lying on her sofa dead that she died of a pulmonary embolism?" asked reporter Cynthia McFadden.

"That's absolutely so," I said. "There is no way that anybody can look at a body and make a diagnosis of a pulmonary embolism. It is not possible."

Pulmonary emboli are blood clots that eventually get trapped in the pulmonary arteries leading to the lungs. Most, about 95 percent, form in the deep veins of the legs, usually in the upper calf, behind the knee, or in the lower thigh. What commonly happens is the clot breaks off, travels through the venous system, which is the veins in a person's body, and into the right side of the heart. From there, the clot will flow to the lungs through the pulmonary artery. That's where it usually becomes obstructed. The results can range from impeded blood flow to instant death.

But this is an internal process. There are no visual clues that scream out blood clot. That could explain why, according to the *New England Journal of Medicine*, 40 percent of pulmonary emboli are not diagnosed correctly. They're hard to evaluate clinically. Sometimes doctors incorrectly believe someone has suffered a heart attack, and the only way to know for sure is to conduct a detailed examination of the heart and lungs. This can be accomplished through specific diagnostic studies if the patient is alive, but in a death case, a careful and thorough autopsy is required to make the diagnosis.

Without an autopsy, one could never know for sure. To me, a postmortem examination was the clearest opportunity to answer once and for all what happened to the country music legend. Richey declined the TV program's request for an interview, but the medical examiner did speak. Dr. Levy acknowledged he couldn't be sure Wynette died of a blood clot in her lungs. He was convinced, however, she died of natural causes.

The night Wynette died, Dr. Levy received a phone call from an investigator on his staff. By that time, a homicide detective had already examined the scene and Wynette's body. The detective found no signs of trauma or foul play. Police also spoke with Dr. Marsh, who told them of Wynette's medical problems that included a "small bowel dysmotility." Based on what he heard that night, Dr. Levy decided not to assume jurisdiction in the case. However, he left instructions for Dr. Marsh to contact the medical examiner's office once he arrived in Nashville and provide his opinion on Wynette's death.

Dr. Levy spoke with Dr. Marsh the next morning. Dr. Marsh told him about Wynette's intestinal dysmotility, which had caused problems related to her getting adequate nutrition and to her developing blood clots. Wynette's past medical history included a hysterectomy and subsequent abdominal surgeries. She also had battled an addiction to painkillers in the late seventies and in the eighties. Since Wynette had suffered through previous clots, Dr.

Marsh told Dr. Levy that he believed one led to her death. The medical examiner found Dr. Marsh's opinion to be reasonable and credible, and stuck with his original decision not to order an autopsy.

By the time Dr. Levy appeared on *20/20*, he already had met with Wynette's daughters and listened to their concerns about the cause of her death and the drugs she had been given to control her pain. "In the last years, I don't know what she was taking, but if they do an autopsy, they will most definitely find several different kinds of narcotics in her," one of Wynette's daughters, Jackie Daly, told the Associated Press in early February.[2]

I can imagine Dr. Levy was surprised to learn that Dr. Marsh never told him or police about three powerful narcotics Wynette was taking when she died. Dr. Marsh said it was a miscommunication between the police and him, a line Dr. Levy repeated during his television interview. But privately, as he later wrote in a report, Dr. Levy suspected there may have been an attempt to provide minimal information to officials the night Wynette died.[3]

The strongest drug Wynette received in the months before her death, through a catheter in her back, was hydromorphone, known as Dilaudid, an analgesic in the same family as morphine and Demerol. It can kill someone in the same way morphine or heroin can, by depressing the brain and thereby causing respiratory and cardiac arrest. The others were midazolam, or Versed, a kind of anesthetic tranquilizer administered during short-term medical procedures; and promethazine, or Phenergan, a mild painkiller. In fact, nine vials of Versed were delivered to Wynette's home the day she died.

As a coroner, knowing that information from the outset would have been critical. I instruct all my deputies to get a full list of medications someone was on at the time of death. Coroners and medical examiners need to have all the facts before being able to decide whether an autopsy is warranted.

Less than two months after the *20/20* segment aired—and almost exactly a year after Tammy Wynette died—her daughters filed a $50-million wrongful-death lawsuit against Richey, Dr. Marsh, and the University of Pittsburgh Medical Center, where Dr. Marsh worked. The lawsuit alleged Dr. Marsh overprescribed medications to Wynette and didn't keep a close enough eye on her condition. It further charged Richey with not getting medical care for Wynette the day that she died.

At about the same time the lawsuit was filed, Pittsburgh attorney Wilbur Otto contacted me. Otto, known as Joe, did legal work for the medical center. He was defending UPMC and Dr. Marsh against the lawsuit brought by Wynette's daughters and wanted to know if I could consult on the case. I had worked on previous cases with Otto, sometimes on the other side, and considered him a very competent and experienced trial attorney. I told him I was willing but immediately raised the issue of the comments I had made on *20/20*. Otto said it would not be a problem.

"Joe, the first thing is you've got to dig up the body and have an autopsy done," I said to him. "It's the right thing to do medically, it's the right thing to do legally, and it's the right thing to do ethically and procedurally for everybody's sake—the husband, the daughters, the medical examiner, and your clients."

Otto agreed, and I offered to conduct the examination if necessary. A week later I learned that wouldn't be needed. Wynette's husband changed his position regarding an autopsy and requested that Dr. Levy conduct one. Authorities exhumed Wynette from her family tomb at Woodlawn Memorial Park in Nashville early on the morning of April 14, 1999. I received a fax from Otto later that morning at roughly the same time Dr. Levy was performing the autopsy. "Had we had more advanced notice of this autopsy being done today, I would have preferred to have you present," Otto wrote.

Although I also would have liked to have been there for the examination, I didn't believe Dr. Levy purposely excluded me. I had been to the Nashville medical examiner's office before, to observe the autopsy of James Earl Ray. Ray, of course, had spent the last thirty years of his life in prison for the killing of Dr. Martin Luther King Jr. After Ray's death in April 1998, his family asked me to witness his autopsy to make sure he died of hepatitis C, as authorities said. During that visit, Dr. Levy was very courteous and I'm sure he would not have objected to my presence in the Wynette case.

In the afternoon, after the autopsy was complete, Richey held a news conference and lashed out at his stepdaughters. He said they had violated their mother's privacy.

"I'm saddened that, out of frustration over financial matters, her daughters have been willing to work so hard to discredit their mother. And that's what they have done," Richey told reporters in a statement. "I'm saddened that part of Tammy's legacy is this fiasco." He requested the autopsy, he said, to "clarify for everyone how Tammy died so we can all move on."[4]

Richey did not answer questions, but his spokeswoman told the gathered media that Richey called Dr. Marsh on April 5—the day before Wynette died—to tell him she seemed sick. Dr. Marsh suggested Richey bring Wynette for medical care. But Wynette refused, saying she was feeling better. Three weeks after Richey requested the autopsy, Wynette's daughters dropped him as a defendant in their lawsuit.

But the case against Dr. Marsh and UPMC continued. Dr. Levy's autopsy findings and results of the toxicology tests could play an important role in determining how far the lawsuit went. The medical examiner did not announce his findings immediately. Rather, he waited until the toxicology tests were completed to offer the full picture of what caused Tammy Wynette's death.

On May 20, 1999, Dr. Levy released his report and conclusions during a press conference with reporters. I eagerly awaited my copy of the document and read through the sixteen pages when they arrived on the fax machine. On the cover page of his autopsy report, Dr. Levy listed as probable cause of death "heart failure with cardiac arrhythmia" due to "chronic pulmonary emboli with pulmonary hypertension." A contributing cause was "intestinal dysmotility on chronic pain management." As for manner of death (homicide, suicide, accident, natural, etc.), Levy marked "could not be determined."

Also included in the materials was a four-paragraph statement from Dr. Levy that he referred to during his press conference. In it, he explained in close to layman's terms what caused Wynette's cardiac arrhythmia, or irregular heartbeat. Dr. Levy said that the right side of her heart had become dilated and enlarged. He concluded that previous blood clots compromised the arteries in Wynette's lungs and caused pressure on the heart's right side as it pushed blood through those obstructions. That then led to the fatal arrhythmia.

I found the diagnosis strange. An arrhythmia is not something you can see or touch. It's a dynamic physiological occurrence that can only be diagnosed in someone alive, whose heart is beating and who is hooked up to an electrocardiogram machine. Alternately, a stethoscope can be used to listen to the heartbeat. Of course, when a patient is dead, that's impossible. Still, however, I didn't believe Dr. Levy's conclusion was implausible or illogical. Most people who die of natural causes will have some sort of arrhythmia, so in a sense such a diagnosis is almost always correct. But you can never be sure.

I also was struck by what Dr. Levy did not find. Despite Dr. Marsh's opinion that Wynette died from a pulmonary embolism, the medical examiner found no acute, that is recent, blood clots in her cardiovascular system. So that was not what caused her death.

Dr. Levy did discover during his microscopic examination that some of Wynette's pulmonary arteries were almost completely obstructed by mature fibrous tissue, or scar tissue. To me, that showed evidence of previous thromboemboli, clots that came from somewhere else in the body and became enlarged once they lodged in her pulmonary artery.

But people don't die from previous thromboemboli. The body adapts. And as far as I could tell from Dr. Levy's description of Wynette's heart, it was essentially normal. The fact that the right ventricle (second chamber) of her heart was markedly dilated does not in and of itself mean anything. It can suggest that blood was not flowing easily and smoothly from the right ventricle to the pulmonary arteries, but there's no proof of that.

I also was interested in the results of the toxicology reports. Dr. Levy had warned back in April when he did the autopsy that, while tests may be able to determine which drugs were in Wynette's system, there was a chance the levels of those drugs would never be known. Three laboratories conducted separate tests for three drugs: Versed, Phenergan, and Dilaudid. The testing revealed the presence of two drugs in Wynette's body when she died: Versed and Phenergan. There was no sign of Dilaudid, the most powerful drug that Wynette had been taking. Unfortunately for everyone involved, embalming fluid breaks down and destroys certain drugs and toxic substances. Dilaudid is one of the substances that dissipates during the embalming process.

In his statement to the press, Dr. Levy said, "It is virtually impossible to determine the exact drug levels of Versed or Phenergan present at the time of Ms. Wynette's death or to what extent, if any, these drugs contributed to her heart failure and death."

I read that and then went back to what Dr. Levy had listed as a contributing cause of death: intestinal dysmotility on chronic pain management. It was another interesting diagnosis, one I have rarely seen. The word *dysmotility* can be broken down into two parts: *dys*, meaning something of an abnormal nature, and *motility*, meaning movement. With that can come abdominal discomfort—at times quite severe—and intermittent episodes of constipation and diarrhea.

It is not uncommon for people who've had abdominal surgery to suffer such symptoms, causing chronic pain, and Wynette had undergone several such operations in the past. When viewing

Wynette's digestive system, Dr. Levy found her stomach, small intestine, and large intestine were matted together with fibrous adhesions. Fibrous tissue is formed as part of the healing process following abdominal surgery. In some instances, that fibrous (scar) tissue can form bands between loops of the intestine and cause sporadic discomfort. Sometimes these bands may actually lead to an intestinal obstruction and require emergency surgery. They also can lead to a perforation of the bowel with infection or obstruction of the bowel, both of which can eventually cause death. But in Wynette's case, there were no obstructions, perforations, or infarctions—segments of the bowel that would have died because of inadequate blood supply. So while these adhesions no doubt caused Wynette pain, they almost certainly didn't contribute directly to her death.

However, Dr. Levy's diagnosis contains the key phrase "chronic pain management." The inference I drew was that perhaps the medical examiner wanted to get across that the drugs Wynette was taking to control her pain—Dilaudid and Versed—played a role in her death. Since he couldn't test for the levels or even determine whether Dilaudid was present, Dr. Levy could not come right out and make such a statement.

Some time after Dr. Levy released his autopsy report, my participation in the case ended. Although I had reviewed all the records and was prepared to testify, a Tennessee law stopped me. The statute prohibits medical experts who are not from Tennessee or one of the geographically contiguous states from testifying in medical malpractice cases. I recommended to Joe Otto that he contact a forensic pathologist from Kentucky, who then joined the defense team.

Meanwhile, George Richey decided to speak at length with *20/20*, the same forum in which three of Wynette's daughters raised questions about his role in Wynette's death. The interview aired January 14, 2000. Richey recounted finding his wife dead on a sofa, where they had been napping the evening of April 6, 1998.

Instead of calling 911, he called Dr. Marsh. "I said, 'She's gone. She's gone. Should I call 911?' And he said, 'Go back and check again.' And I checked again. And I went back to the phone and I said, 'She is gone, Wallis, she is gone.' And he said, 'No, there's no reason to call 911.'"

Richey went on to say Dr. Marsh signed Wynette's death certificate because her local doctor was out of town. His objection to an autopsy stemmed from statements he said his wife often made to him: she did not want to be cremated and did not want an autopsy. Richey denied accusations by Wynette's daughters that he over-medicated her against her will and said Wynette sometimes gave herself injections. The *20/20* correspondent, Cynthia McFadden, asked more questions about Dr. Marsh and his actions, prompting Richey to come to the doctor's defense.

"Let me make it very clear, I have never met a more committed surgeon and physician than Dr. Wallis Marsh," Richey said. "So, I give him credit, not only with magnificent treatment, but extending her life, not contributing to her death."

Dr. Marsh declined the program's request for an interview, citing the pending lawsuit. But his attorneys had already released a statement within days of the case being filed back in April 1999. In it, they said that when the facts came out, it would be clear that Dr. Marsh and other physicians at UPMC who worked on a treatment plan "provided extraordinary medical care to a person who suffered extraordinary medical problems."

Even as Richey talked with *20/20*, the daughters' case continued on in federal court. Though Richey had been dropped as a defendant, Wynette's daughters added Care Solutions of Nashville, a pharmacy that supplied Wynette prescriptions. The pharmacy should have questioned the amount of medications Dr. Marsh was prescribing, the daughters charged.

But in the end there was no trial. U.S. District Judge Todd

Campbell dismissed the case against Care Solutions in October 2001. Six months later, Wynette's daughters and Dr. Marsh reached a settlement. The terms were confidential.

Before the case ended, medical examiner Dr. Levy also made a finding that cleared up lingering questions. He changed the manner of Wynette's death from "could not be determined" to "natural causes." Dr. Levy made the revision after reviewing evidence provided by Otto and other attorneys for Dr. Marsh. The evidence consisted of newly published research regarding the breakdown of Versed as it reacts with embalming fluid. The result is a product unique from the original, Dr. Levy said.

He noted Versed was found by just one of the three labs that did the initial testing of samples from Wynette. Subsequent testing by two more labs chosen by Dr. Marsh's attorneys also failed to reveal the drug's presence in the samples. Based on the new research and that four out of five laboratories returned negative results, Dr. Levy concluded that the positive result should be discounted. Under the circumstances, this seemed to me like an appropriate decision.

In my mind, much time and effort was spent and unnecessary anguish suffered by many people in this case. Much, if not all of it, could have been spared had Dr. Marsh provided a full accounting of the drugs Wynette was taking and had Dr. Levy ordered an immediate autopsy. That way, all the facts would have been up front and available for anyone to evaluate. But that didn't happen. So to this day, I am not sure why Tammy Wynette died. It may have occurred the way Dr. Levy suggests—the right side of her heart became enlarged and that caused a fatal cardiac arrhythmia. But there's just no way to prove his analysis scientifically.

Some answers about the death of one of country music's greatest female singers may never be known.

Chapter Seven

THE TRIALS OF O. J.

The Final Verdict

I N THE WINTER OF 1997, A Los Angeles jury filed into a packed courtroom. Their charge was clear: determine if O. J. Simpson was responsible for the deaths of his ex-wife, Nicole Brown Simpson, and her friend, Ronald Lyle Goldman. For forty-one days, lawyers on both sides had presented reams of evidence, sworn testimony, oral arguments, and theatrics.

The twelve-person jury heard from 101 witnesses. More than 2,500 exhibits or pieces of evidence were given to the panel to examine. They had been lectured for weeks about DNA fingerprinting, blood splatters, autopsies, and crime scene evidence. For two days they deliberated. Their mission was to decide which side was telling the truth. Did the former football star and television commentator kill the pair in a fit of rage and then attempt to cover it up? Or were the police guilty of framing O. J. for the murders and planting evidence against him?

On February 4, 1997, the panel entered the courtroom to deliver their unanimous verdict. Many people were shocked at how quickly the dozen men and women of the jury had reviewed the evidence, considered the testimony, and come to a conclusion. But the jurors were certain and in total agreement about their decision.

Once they were all seated, the judge asked if they had reached a verdict. The foreman of the jury rose from his chair.

"We have, Your Honor," he responded.

The juror handed the courtroom bailiff the verdict forms. They were passed on to the judge for his review. After only a few seconds of skimming the official verdict form, the judge had the court officer return the form to the jury foreman. With cameras focused, reporters jotting down every sigh and smile, the foreman of the jury announced their decision.

It was, as Yogi Berra once put it, déjà vu all over again.

Just eighteen months earlier, a separate jury had tackled this same task. They, too, had been asked to consider O. J.'s guilt in the murders. That first jury had seen 126 people take the witness stand. More than 1,000 pieces of evidence had been handed to them during a trial that lasted an amazing thirty-three weeks. That first jury had also done its job under the microscope of national media attention.

Both cases were tried in Los Angeles with California jurors weighing the evidence. The allegations in each case were the same, the two juries were presented essentially the same evidence, and the same witnesses testified. Yet the results in the two cases were a study in contrast. The first jury cleared O. J. of all charges. The second jury found him responsible for the deaths of his ex-wife and her friend.

As the years pass, most of the highest profile trials fade from view, yet the O. J. Simpson case continues to be one of the most memorable public events of our time—right up there with the assassination of President John F. Kennedy, the explosion of the space shuttle *Challenger*, and the terrorist attacks of September 11.

Whenever I speak to law or medical organizations or to various community groups, I am almost always asked my thoughts on the guilt of O. J. And one question that constantly arises is: How could the jury in the first trial find O. J. innocent while the second jury find him guilty? And that question is usually followed by: Why was O. J. put on trial twice? Isn't that double jeopardy?

The questions reflect the public's continuing fascination with the case. But both questions also show that there is a basic misunderstanding of our laws and our civil and criminal justice systems. To me, the O. J. case provides the perfect opportunity to explain to people the workings of our legal system, as well as the chance to showcase advances in forensic sciences.

The short answer is that while the two trials sought to find the same truth—whether O. J. Simpson killed Nicole Brown Simpson and Ronald Goldman—based on virtually the same evidence, they are two very different proceedings. Not only is it legally acceptable that the two juries reached different verdicts, but also, I believe both juries reached the technically correct decision in their respective cases.

That said, I want to make one point very clear: neither case successfully exposed the complete truth regarding what happened the night of June 12, 1994, outside the home of Nicole Simpson. Trials are about advocacy, following rules of evidence, proving specific allegations, and meeting certain constitutional requirements or burdens. Trials are not necessarily about seeking and determining the truth.

But, as the fictitious FBI agent Fox Mulder on the television drama *The X-Files* frequently proclaimed, "The truth is out there." In cases like this, the truth about what really happened can be found in the forensic science and legal-medical investigations. The truth about how Nicole and Ronald Goldman died, as exposed by the scientific evidence in this case, is very different from the story told by the lawyers at either trial. The truth in this case lies in the blood spatters on dirty socks, in the angle of the deadly stab wounds, and in barely noticed footprints on a pair of pants.

To better understand what really occurred on June 12, 1994, at 875 South Bundy Drive and why the truth wasn't revealed in either trial, it is important to examine the background and facts of the two cases.

The combination of high-profile and colorful characters, legal complexities, sensational allegations from both sides, extensive media coverage, and constant public attention clearly made the case of O. J. Simpson one of the most infamous trials of the twentieth century. Many murder cases gain notoriety in the press, but most of the time the attention begins to wane after a few days or weeks. That simply wasn't so with this case. From day one, the investigation into the murders of Nicole Brown Simpson and Ron Goldman commanded nonstop coverage from the news media and the general public, who had an insatiable appetite to hear as much as possible about the case. If anything, public fascination and media scrutiny increased every day as the case progressed. The public was so consumed with the matter that by the time the case went to trial six months later, the television networks frequently broke away from their normal programming of soap operas to broadcast testimony live from the Los Angeles courtroom.

Why?

There are several answers. First, the case had all the key elements that make up a movie thriller. The focus of the case was a poor young man who had worked hard to become a beloved athlete, network television announcer, and movie star. The supporting characters were colorful, dramatic, and bizarre, including house guest Kato Kaelin, Los Angeles police detective Mark Fuhrman, prosecutors Marcia Clark and Christopher Darden, defense lawyers Johnnie Cochran and F. Lee Bailey, and Judge Lance Ito.

The crime of which O. J. was accused was truly heinous. The case itself contained many mysteries, with some evidence pointing toward guilt and other evidence seemingly supporting Simpson's innocence. Serious allegations of police misconduct and fabrication of evidence contributed to the drama. There was also the issue of race—a black husband accused of killing his young, beautiful, blonde, white ex-wife in Los Angeles. It was heightened by the fact that it occurred in the wake of the Rodney King fiasco. Add to this the money factor—that O. J. lived in the elite Brentwood community and that he had the wealth to hire the best lawyers to help him fight the charges.

And, of course, there were the surreal elements—from the bizarre low-speed Bronco ride and police chase to the wailing dog at the crime scene. Greta Van Susteren, now a commentator on Fox, described the case to me as a "great trash novel come to life." The *Dallas Morning News* on December 19, 1995, reported that when Russian president Boris Yeltsin visited with President Bill Clinton in 1995, his first question was: "Do you think O. J. did it?"

Finally, the media played a major role in securing O. J. Simpson's case in history. In some respects, the news media simply feeds a public thirst for information. There's a legitimate argument that the press would not have focused as much on the O. J. case if their viewers, readers, and listeners didn't want them to. The case provided amazing, real-life entertainment and drama for which people hunger. And there's no disputing that O. J. and the case were newsworthy.

That being said, the media clearly went overboard in its continuous coverage. In 1994, national cable news programs, including CNBC and CNN, were seeing their ratings or viewership skyrocket. Just like twenty-four-hour talk-radio stations, these cable television news networks had to fill their airtime with some kind of programming. Until O. J., these shows covered stories on futuristic mass transit systems, oil exploration in Alaska, or how much vodka Russian president Boris Yeltsin drank by noon every day—worthy subjects to be sure, but none as fascinating—or at least not as sensational—as the "trial of the century."

However, people should not dismiss the Simpson case as a complete aberration in our nation's legal history. To do so would be to bury one of the fiercest and most fascinating court battles of all time. If ever there was a case in the history of jurisprudence that should be analyzed and studied by law professors, criminal justice experts, court officials, bar associations, and laymen around the country, it is the O. J. Simpson murder case.

From the moment the bodies were discovered to the skirmishes in court that probably continue to this day, the Simpson court file raises a multitude of fascinating legal, societal, and moral issues. The case can be used to examine what it means to receive a fair trial under the Sixth Amendment to the U.S. Constitution, or the right to be judged by a jury of your peers, or the right to be considered innocent until proven guilty, or the constitutional burden placed on the state or the government to prove someone's guilt beyond a reasonable doubt. There are also broader debates raised by the matter, including the value of human life or the ability of the wealthy to essentially buy their way out of trouble.

My involvement in the Simpson case was twofold. First, several of the lawyers and expert witnesses hired by O. J. for the criminal case are close friends and colleagues of mine. Individually and together, I consulted with them by phone and in person about the Simpson case. For example, trial lawyer F. Lee Bailey, who has been a personal friend of mine for many years, came to Pittsburgh to get my advice on which expert witnesses to call to testify. Simpson's DNA legal specialist Barry Scheck and I have worked together on many cases, as have I and Harvard law professor Alan Dershowitz.

Four highly experienced forensic scientists were key witnesses for the defense. Dr. Michael Baden, the codirector of the New York

State Police Forensic Sciences Unit, testified about the autopsies, the time of death, and the manner in which the victims were attacked. Dr. Henry Lee, the director of the Connecticut State Police Forensic Laboratory, testified about the crime scene and DNA testing. Herb MacDonell, the director of the Laboratory of Forensic Science in Corning, New York, testified about the physical evidence. And Dr. Fredric Rieders, director of the National Medical Services (a highly respected toxicology lab based in Willow Grove, Pennsylvania), testified about the alcohol levels in the victims' blood.

Throughout the case, I spoke with each of these experts regularly about the evidence. Not that any of them needed my help or advice, of course; they are the most preeminent forensic scientists in the world. But they are also my friends, so they would call me to talk through ideas or thoughts or to gauge my response to something. However, I was never a paid consultant for the defense. I reviewed the defense's evidence, including autopsy and crime scene reports, for free.

That allowed me to pursue my second involvement in this case without any strings attached—being a commentator or analyst on the case for NBC, ABC, and CNN. If I had accepted money from Simpson or his defense team for my assistance, I would have felt a professional obligation as a hired expert witness to refrain from criticizing evidence or arguments presented by Simpson's legal team. That doesn't mean I would alter my opinion or lie about my view just because I'm a hired consultant. It does mean I would have been an advocate for Simpson's side of the case.

The bottom line is that I did not want any possible conflicts of interest. I wanted to be able to tell Tom Brokaw or Larry King what I really thought, even if it was damaging to O. J. I wanted to be able to examine and comment on the evidence and legal arguments without feeling any restrictions. I wanted to analyze this case without fear or favor.

The first step in understanding the public intrigue in the Simpson case is to grasp the amazing life of O. J. himself and how he overcame so many obstacles to become so successful and respected.

Orenthal James Simpson was born in San Francisco in 1947 to Eunice and Jimmy Lee Simpson. The man who would become known as "the Juice" and who would become famous worldwide for his athletic prowess had a rocky start in life. When he was a few months old, his parents noticed that something was wrong with his legs. Doctors diagnosed him with rickets—a vitamin D deficiency that weakens and disturbs the growth of the bones. The physicians' proposed solution was to surgically break the small boy's legs and reset them with braces. But the Simpsons were poor, so they rejected the surgery. Instead young O. J. wore a homemade brace with special shoes that his parents forced him to wear on the wrong feet. Other grade-school students gave O. J. a nickname—"Pencil Pins"—because his legs were so long and thin, though the braces had made him bowlegged.

Simpson poured himself into athletics because he was a below-average student. By middle school, an amazing thing happened: O. J. discovered the braces had worked. He could run as fast as the other boys. Socializing became another priority for Simpson. In high school his outgoing and friendly personality placed him in positions of leadership. He was head of a group called "the Superiors," which organized school dances and community projects for young people. In sharp contrast, however, O. J. also led the "Persian Warriors," a street gang that specialized in stealing and drinking.

It was those types of antics that landed O. J. in juvenile court at age fifteen. When he went home to face his parents, instead of his father waiting to lecture him, there stood Willie Mays. The all-star outfielder for the San Francisco Giants was a friend of Simpson's football coach. Hearing of his athletic promise, Mays agreed to try to help set him straight. The Hall of Fame athlete talked to the teenager for a while before taking the youngster to his own home in one of the wealthiest sections of town.

Family and friends say that it was seeing how Mays lived in luxury that inspired O. J. to clean up his act. He decided to make sports, especially football, his ticket to wealth and fame. Galileo High School, which O. J. attended, wasn't known for being a football powerhouse, but that changed during Simpson's senior year. One of their first games of the season was against St. Ignatius, a team that had beaten them the last twenty-three games. For the first half, it looked as if game twenty-four would go in the same direction, with St. Ignatius leading by a blistering 25-10. Then O. J. took control and scored touchdowns on sixty-, eighty-, and ninety-yard runs. St. Ignatius's coach was so dazzled that night that he called a friend who was an assistant coach for the University of Southern California Trojans.

USC immediately sent scouts to Galileo High's games. They were equally impressed, and Simpson was placed at the top of their recruiting agenda. But there was a barrier: O. J.'s poor grades had caught up with him. USC let him know they were very interested in him but he needed to attend a junior college for two years to raise his scores.

Two years later, in 1965, O. J.'s grades had improved, so the university kept its promise of a full football scholarship. Simpson quickly broke almost every USC rushing record. In 1968 he won the Heisman Trophy, which recognizes the best college football player in the country.

The next year, the Buffalo Bills, the team with the worst record in the National Football League, made O. J. Simpson the first player chosen in the annual draft. For a decade, Simpson swept away fans of professional football. He found holes in defensive lines like no other running back in history had done. I remember watching him play against the Detroit Lions one Thanksgiving in the early seventies. That was the day he set the single-game rushing record. It seemed like he could change direction in midair. And his record crunching went on. In 1973 he set the single-season rushing record with 2,003 yards—especially incredible when one considers the less-than-stellar team for which he played. Many football analysts feel that Simpson had the potential to be the greatest football player of all time if he had played for one of the top teams of the era such as the Miami Dolphins.

But football was rough on the man who had started life in braces. By the late seventies, his knees began to give out. I remember an article that quoted Simpson saying he was so sore, bruised, and beaten up after a Sunday game that he couldn't even practice again until Thursday. Finally, in 1978, the Juice hung up his cleats and looked around to see what else life had to offer.

During his football career, O. J. had developed a reputation with the public and his friends for being one of the nicest guys around. He donated much of his time to projects for needy children. He never turned away or charged for autographs, and his generosity to charities was almost to a fault. This "good-guy" image, combined with Simpson's ambition, guaranteed him smooth sailing into the world of media, movies, and corporate America.

O. J.'s national reputation had been enhanced when he was seen on television commercials, on billboards, and in magazine advertisements running and leaping through airports to catch a plane after Hertz Rental Car company made him their national spokesperson. Upon his retirement from the NFL, he was signed by ABC, and later NBC, to be a commentator on pro football games. He further expanded his portfolio and the love of his fans when he acted in such popular films as *The Towering Inferno* and the *Naked Gun* series.

Simpson's personal life seemed charmed. He earned more

money than he ever believed possible. He was famous, recognized everywhere he went. The best restaurants provided him instant seating. Unlike many black athletes before him, O. J. easily crossed racial barriers. While playing pro football, he married his high-school sweetheart. The couple had three children—two daughters and a son.

But Simpson's life took a dramatic turn in 1980 when tragedy visited his family. Aaren, his twenty-three-month-old daughter, died when she accidentally drowned in the family's swimming pool. The traumatic event exposed cracks in the couple's marriage and flaws in the American hero's reputation. Rumors of drug use surfaced. His wife filed for divorce, claiming O. J. was a womanizer. And stories about Simpson's temper also emerged, though mainly in the tabloids.

A couple of years earlier, Simpson had met a tall, beautiful teenager, Nicole Brown. She was eighteen and a waitress at Daisy's, a Beverly Hills nightclub frequented by O. J. They dated publicly for several years and finally married in 1985. They were constantly spotted around town at the trendiest dance clubs. His annual income from being a sports commentator, his movie gigs, and commercial endorsements was estimated to be about $700,000 a year. His net worth, according to one report, topped $10 million. They owned million-dollar houses in tony Brentwood, beautiful Laguna Beach, and popular Manhattan Beach. Together they had two children.

In 1992, O. J. and Nicole divorced. There were allegations—mostly in the tabloid press—about spousal abuse. Yet Simpson's reputation remained sterling.

Then came the night of June 12, 1994. Nicole returned to her condominium at 875 South Bundy Drive about 9:35 P.M. She, her mother, and her father had been to dinner. Minutes after Nicole had taken off her coat, her mother, Judith Brown, called saying she had left her sunglasses at Mezzaluna's, the trendy Los Angeles restaurant where they had eaten. Nicole reminded her mother that she knew the waiter at the restaurant and would call him to see if anyone had found the glasses.

Nicole immediately called Mezzaluna's. The waiter, Ron Goldman, quickly spotted the glasses and promised to bring them by Nicole's condo on his way home that evening. It won't be long, he told her on the phone, because he was about to finish work. Fellow employees said he left for Nicole's home about 9:50 P.M.

About midnight a couple who lived down the street from Nicole were walking their dog when they spotted Nicole's Akita wandering the streets. The dog, whose paws were bloodied, immediately led them back to Nicole's condo, where the couple discovered the bodies and then called the police.

Like most others, I heard about the murders the next morning on television. The crimes had occurred too late to make the morning newspapers. And details were sketchy even on TV. My first thoughts were simple: Where was O. J.? Was he responsible? After four decades of investigating bizarre murders, I immediately think about possible suspects. Spouses are always prime suspects at the beginning of such cases.

The fact that the murders were stabbings indicated that the crimes were very personal. My forty-plus years as a medicolegal investigator taught me that slayings involving a knife are much more intense and intimate than homicides involving a gun. It's much easier to stand back at a distance and pull a trigger. In fact, the victim doesn't even have to see the assailant in a shooting. But to commit a stabbing requires a perpetrator to stand extremely close, probably even face the victim. And the fact that the attacker's hands are connected to the knife that is plunging into the victim, probably even touching the victim, makes stabbings more likely to be committed by someone who is extremely angry at the victim.

Initially I was relieved when I heard that Simpson was in Chicago at the O'Hare Plaza Hotel for a golf tournament sponsored by Hertz when he learned of his ex-wife's homicide. Like everyone who admired O. J.'s athletic accomplishments, I wanted him to be cleared of any wrongdoing.

Simpson, who was forty-six years old at the time, immediately flew home to be with his children. Los Angeles police detectives, who wanted Simpson to answer some questions, met him at LAX. The former football star agreed to talk to the police and said he didn't need or want a lawyer to be present.

The next afternoon, June 13, O. J. met with Detectives Philip Vannatter and Thomas Lange at a police station near Simpson's home. After reading O. J. his *Miranda* rights, the two investigators queried Simpson for about thirty minutes. I was provided a transcribed copy of the interview by lawyers involved in the case.

Simpson said he had seen Nicole the evening before, June 12, about 6:30 P.M., at a dance recital for the couple's daughter, Sydney. For several minutes, they had O. J. walk them through his day and evening. The detectives asked how he had received a cut on his right hand. Simpson claimed he was holding a glass in his hotel room when police called to inform him of the murders.

"I just kind of went bonkers for a little bit," he said.

"Is that how you cut it?" Lange inquired.

"It was cut before, but I think I just opened it again," Simpson answered. "I'm not sure."

"Do you recall bleeding at all in your truck, in the Bronco?" Lange asked.

"I recall bleeding at my house, and then I went to the Bronco," Simpson responded. "The last thing I did before I left, when I was rushing, was went and got my phone out of the Bronco."

"So, do you recall bleeding at all?" Lange asked.

"Yeah, I mean, I knew I was bleeding, but it was no big deal."

Simpson said. "I play golf and stuff, so there's always something, nicks and stuff, here and there."

"You haven't had any problems with Nicole lately, have you?" Vannatter inquired.

"I always have problems with her, you know," Simpson answered. "Our relationship has been a problem relationship."

"Did Nicole have words with you last night?" Vannatter asked.

"No, not at all," Simpson said.

"O. J., we've got sort of a problem," Vannatter stated. "We've got some blood on your car. We've got some blood at your house, and sort of a problem."

"Well, take my blood test," Simpson immediate spoke up.

"Well, we'd like to do that," Lange said. "We've got, of course, the cut on your finger that you aren't real clear on. Do you recall having that cut on your finger the last time you were at Nicole's house?"

"A week ago?" Simpson asked.

"Yeah."

"No," Simpson responded. "It was cut last night."

Then Detective Vannatter went straight to the heart of the case. "What do you think happened? Do you have any idea?"

"I have no idea, man," Simpson answered. "You guys haven't told me anything. I have absolutely no idea what happened. I don't know how, why, or what. But you guys haven't told me anything. Every time I ask you guys, you say you're going to tell me in a bit."

"Did you ever hit her, O. J.?" Vannatter asked.

"One night, we had a fight," Simpson said. "We had a fight and she hit me. And they never took my statement. They never wanted to hear my side and they never wanted to hear my housekeeper's side. Nicole was drunk. She did her thing and started tearing up my house, you know. I didn't punch or anything, but I . . ."

"Slapped her a couple times," Vannatter injected.

"No, no," Simpson quickly answered. "I wrestled her, is what I did. I didn't slap her at all."

"Understand, the reason we're talking to you is because you're the ex-husband," Lange said.

"I know I'm the number-one target, and now you tell me I've got blood all over the place," Simpson said.

Thirty-two minutes later the police interview ended. A police photographer took a few snapshots of the cuts on O. J.'s hands and then the police released him.

News that Simpson had cooperated with police and answered their questions was quickly leaked to the media. It was also announced that Simpson had consented to a complete search of his home. Many commentators said this indicated either that Simpson had nothing to hide or that he made a very stupid mistake. Famous people often think they can talk their way out of trouble or explain away issues, so they frequently waive their Fifth Amendment right against self-incrimination and agree to talk to police or answer questions from a grand jury that is investigating criminal activity. The bigger the ego, the more likely this is to happen. The problem is that authorities usually have the answers to their questions before they even ask them. The prosecutors or police are simply seeing if the witness will lie.

All that being said, Simpson's decision to talk to police immediately worked out well for him for two reasons. First, he didn't say anything incriminating. Second, the detectives' questions were extremely benign. So weak was this interview that prosecutors refused to introduce it to the jury during the trial.

The next time the public saw Simpson was two days later, June 16, at Nicole's funeral. He held his children's hands. He hugged friends. All the police would say publicly is that "no one has been ruled out" as suspects.

But behind the scenes, authorities had decided O. J. was their man. Late that night, prosecutors contacted Simpson's lawyer, Robert Shapiro, to say they were indeed going to arrest O. J. for the two murders. Shapiro said Simpson would voluntarily turn himself in to police the next morning at ten. Reports that O. J. was about to be arrested leaked to the press. It was instantly all over the news.

When Simpson failed to turn himself in to police that morning, the authorities went looking for him. Eventually, they put out an all-points bulletin seeking his arrest.

That night, my wife and I were eating dinner at a restaurant in Pittsburgh. As I walked toward the restroom to wash my hands, I noticed several people standing around the television at the bar. Intrigued, I stopped to see what was so gripping. On the screen was a white Ford Bronco traveling at an amazingly slow speed. Following the Bronco were a dozen or so police cars with their red-and-blue flashing lights turned on. The police cars were one hundred feet or so behind the Bronco, but also traveling at twenty to thirty miles per hour. It was obvious that the officers were making no effort to stop the car or to pull up beside it. The normally packed Los Angeles freeway was completely empty of traffic—except for the handful of cars parked alongside the highway waving their hands or holding signs that read: "We love you, O. J." Circling above the Bronco and police were a multitude of news media helicopters equipped with live camera satellite feeds.

The announcers on television were reporting that Simpson's best friend, Al Cowlings, was driving the Bronco and that O. J. was in the back seat with a gun pointed to his head, threatening to kill himself if the police got any closer. It was truly one of the most surreal scenes ever on American television. And it captivated the attention of Americans, as a reported 95 million people watched the bizarre police chase.

About halfway through O. J.'s freeway marathon, Robert Kardashian, Simpson's personal lawyer, appeared before the television cameras and radio microphones. He began reading a letter O. J. had left behind. It was addressed "To Whom It May Concern" and was widely interpreted as a suicide note.

"I have nothing to do with Nicole's murder," it read. "I loved her, always have and always will. If we had a problem, it's because I loved her so much."

Later in the note, Simpson wrote, "I don't want to belabor knocking the press, but I can't believe what is being said. Most of it is totally made up. I know you have a job to do, but as a last wish, please, please, please, leave my children in peace. Their lives will be tough enough. At times, I have felt like a battered husband or boyfriend, but I loved her, make that clear to everyone."

He concluded the letter with these remarks: "Don't feel sorry for me. I've had a great life, great friends. Please think of the real O. J. and not this lost person. Thanks for making my life special. I hope I helped yours. Peace and love, O. J."

Kardashian then publicly pleaded with O. J. to put down his pistol, stop the Bronco, and turn himself in peacefully. Other members of his family, including Simpson's own mother, also begged Simpson not to harm himself and to end the chase safely for the sake of his children. All the while, police and lawyers were in communication with Cowlings and Simpson via cell phone in an attempt to negotiate a peaceful ending.

As the sun set on California, the Bronco pulled into the driveway of Simpson's Brentwood home. Cowlings exited the vehicle first and was quickly pulled away by police. Then, a minute later, a haggard-looking Simpson appeared. He raised his hands and was quickly surrounded by police. Inside the Bronco, authorities found $8,750 cash, a false beard, a loaded pistol, and a passport.

The next day, NBC called to see if I would do a live interview with Tom Brokaw about the case. I had just arrived at my summer home in New Haven, Connecticut, and told the NBC producer I could do the interview at their studios in New York City, which I did.

During one of the commercial breaks, I received a call from my good friend and colleague Dr. Michael Baden, who, as I mentioned earlier, is the former chief medical examiner for New York City and considered one of the world's leading forensic pathologists. Dr. Baden had told me two days earlier that Shapiro had called him and asked him to fly immediately to Los Angeles to review the case and examine the autopsy findings.

Before I could ask him his thoughts or feelings on the case, Dr. Baden shocked me with the following story that told me what really happened the day O. J. fled. About 11 A.M. Pacific time on June 17, Shapiro had taken Dr. Baden and our good friend and colleague Dr. Henry Lee, the renowned criminalist, to the home of O. J.'s personal lawyer, Robert Kardashian. The lawyer informed Drs. Baden and Lee that Simpson would be arrested and charged with the homicides. But before Simpson was taken into custody, Shapiro wanted them to examine cuts on O. J.'s hands. For several minutes, the duo examined and photographed Simpson's hands. They also took blood and hair samples, in case police and prosecutors would not allow them to do so after Simpson was arrested.

"There are definite cuts, but the cuts are jagged," Dr. Baden told me on the phone. "To me, they are more consistent with O. J.'s story that he cut his hands on a glass at his hotel when he learned of Nicole's murder. The cuts are not consistent with knife wounds."

Dr. Baden said that when Simpson failed to turn himself in at the police station at 10 A.M., authorities called Shapiro. The lawyer told them that Simpson was with him at Kardashian's house. He said they were welcome to meet him there, and O. J. would go with them then.

At 1 P.M., four uniformed officers knocked on Kardashian's front door, according to Dr. Baden. Shapiro answered, inviting the officers inside. He told them Simpson had gone upstairs with his best friend, Al Cowlings. When Shapiro and Kardashian yelled out for Simpson to come downstairs, there was no response. Kardashian walked upstairs to bring Simpson down, but he returned without O. J., saying his client was nowhere to be found.

"Only after about five minutes of searching did it hit us," Dr. Baden told me. "O. J. was gone. He had snuck out."

According to Baden, that alarmed police, who immediately announced that everyone on the premises was under house arrest. "They thought Henry and I had somehow helped O. J. escape."

Fortunately, one of the detectives at the scene spotted Dr. Lee, who is one of the nation's leading experts on DNA testing and crime scene investigations and who is universally respected for his integrity. "When they recognized Henry, they let us go," Dr. Baden said with a sigh of relief.

But Dr. Baden said he was very worried about Simpson's state of mind. He said Simpson answered all his questions, but he did so with very short answers—usually yes or no.

"He seemed very depressed," Dr. Baden said. "He appeared very lethargic and apathetic."

On June 22, Simpson made his first appearance in court. This preliminary hearing was brief and had two purposes. The defendant—Simpson—would officially enter his plea of not guilty or guilty, and it was also the time when a defendant, held in jail, can ask the judge to set a bond so that he can be released. The plea portion of the hearing is formal. Almost never does a defendant plead guilty, unless there has been some prearranged deal with prosecutors.

In this case, the judge asked Simpson how he was pleading to the charges. Simpson rose from his chair: "Absolutely 100 percent not guilty." Defense lawyers did ask the court to set aside time for a probable cause hearing. Shapiro said he planned to challenge the charges immediately by arguing that there was not enough evidence to sustain the charges against his client.

213

During the six days of probable cause hearings, I served as a legal and medical expert for NBC and ABC. I watched the testimony, presentation of evidence, and oral arguments from a studio at Rockefeller Center. Then Tom Brokaw would ask for my interpretation and analysis. In the evenings, I agreed to appear a handful of times on CNN's *Crossfire*, which at the time was hosted by conservative Patrick Buchanan and liberal Michael Kinsley. All the while, I was having private conversations with Drs. Baden and Lee, and F. Lee Bailey, who recently had been hired by Simpson to join his legal defense team.

The hearings ended on July 8 when Judge Kathleen Kennedy-Powell ruled that she found there was probable cause or sufficient evidence to conclude that Simpson might have committed the crimes. Whether the state had enough evidence to prove it beyond a reasonable doubt, she said, would need to be left to a jury to decide. No one, including the strongest supporters of Simpson or his own lawyers, believed the judge would throw out the charges. But it was an excellent opportunity for Simpson's defense lawyers to get a first-hand look at the prosecution's case and the potential flaws in it.

After several intense weeks of courtroom battles over what evidence could and could not be presented to the jury, Judge Lance Ito began the criminal trial, the *State of California* v. *Orenthal James Simpson*, on September 24. The Los Angeles district attorney's office decided to file the murder charges at the downtown district courthouse instead of the Santa Monica district courthouse, which is in Los Angeles County and closer to the scene of the crime. Prosecutors chose to file the case downtown to reduce the commute time of the lawyers handling the high-profile matter and to better accommodate the massive media attention.

Lawyers told me privately that there was another reason, a political motivation. The Santa Monica district where Simpson lived was overwhelmingly white and wealthy. Prosecutors feared a conviction by an all-white jury could spark racial protests, or worse, racial riots. Keep in mind, the Simpson case took place right on the heels of the Rodney King police beating case, in which the officers were acquitted after all of America viewed that troubling video. No question, racial tensions were high. By contrast, the downtown district was more likely to attract largely lower-income and minority citizens to jury service. But prosecutors were confident they had such strong and convincing evidence that they would win a conviction no matter the makeup of the jury.

While many legal experts condemn the prosecutors for deciding to handle the case downtown instead of in Santa Monica, I am not so critical. Would the jury verdict have been different if authorities had tried the charges in Santa Monica? I'm not so sure.

When deciding to prosecute a murder case, district attorneys have to make many choices, many of them with political overtones. Do they file charges at all? Should the charges be first-degree murder or a lesser homicide charge such as manslaughter or second degree? Should they seek the death penalty or life in prison? In which jurisdiction should the charges be filed?

As you will read, I am extremely critical of how prosecutors handled this case. It was their case to lose, and they did a great job losing it. But I will not blast the district attorneys for deciding to file the charges downtown instead of in Santa Monica. A prosecutor's job is to seek justice, not to win at any cost. Yes, prosecutors will try to win convictions, but in a community such as Los Angeles, where racial tensions were so high at the time, the decision about where to try this case had to include a consideration about the racial composition of the jury. I also believe that at the time the prosecutors filed the charges, they looked at the evidence police had gathered and truly believed that they had a slam-dunk case. Prosecutors probably felt they could get a guilty verdict from a jury of the most adamant O. J. supporters.

215

To start the trial, Judge Ito summoned to jury duty more than 250 Los Angeles residents, who were randomly chosen from the California driver's license and voter registration lists. Prosecutors and defense attorneys hired jury consultants to help them decide which questions to ask the potential jurors and which jurors to excuse. Remember, jury selection is more about deselecting or eliminating people from serving on a jury than it is about choosing who should serve. That's because state laws give each side in a trial a certain number of peremptory strikes that the lawyers can use to eliminate people from the jury for any reason other than race or gender.

Lawyers in the Simpson case developed a seventy-nine-page questionnaire with 294 questions about the lives, thoughts, and beliefs of the potential jurors. Prospective jurors were asked about their attitudes toward interracial marriages, domestic abuse, religion, and professional athletes. They were questioned about the books and newspapers they read, the organizations to which they belonged, the churches they attended, and the people whom they considered heroes. It was hoped that requiring the jurors to fill out the written questionnaire would shorten the length of jury selection. Unfortunately, it didn't work out that way. It took five weeks for prosecutors, defense lawyers, and Judge Ito to pick a jury.

In the end, a jury of ten women and two men was chosen. The panel included nine black people, two white people, and one Latino person. Two of them were college graduates. None of them subscribed to a daily newspaper, though eight watched tabloid television shows, such as *Hard Copy* or *A Current Affair*. All were registered Democrats. Five of them said that they or members of their families had previously had negative experiences with police officers. But all twelve promised to put aside any personal prejudices they had and swore they would judge the case solely on the evidence presented during the trial.

The criminal trial lasted an astonishing 133 days. The jurors were sequestered the entire time. Each side took a day for opening statements. The prosecution called seventy-two witnesses during the ninety-nine days it took to present its side of the case. The state's case proved unwieldy and unmanageable. Prosecutors did a poor job of moving their presentation quickly and efficiently. As a result, key evidence was buried or long forgotten by the end of the case.

Even so, it was a truly fascinating case to watch unfold. Both NBC News and CNN regularly asked me to comment on or explain the evidence being presented during the trial. A day seldom passed during the trial when someone from the *Los Angeles Times*, *USA Today*, the Associated Press, ABC Radio News, or some other national news program wouldn't call to get my comments on the case. That is why I had to follow the case very closely. In addition, I was having regular meetings and consultations with key members of the defense team.

The defense team Simpson assembled was an amazing team of lawyers. The news media referred to the group as "the Dream Team," and it consisted of Robert Shapiro, F. Lee Bailey, Johnnie Cochran, and Barry Scheck—all legal heavyweights. Normally, the defense portion of a criminal trial is not very long. That's because defense lawyers seldom have much to add in criminal trials other than to attack the state's evidence or arguments. But the lawyers for Simpson had definite points and messages. They proactively attacked the prosecution's case by calling witnesses to refute key testimony or to put a different twist on evidence. As a result, defense attorneys took from July 10 through September 8 to make their case.

Simpson waived his right to testify in his criminal trial. In doing so, Simpson told Judge Ito that he "did not, could not, and would not have committed this crime."

Closing arguments for each side lasted two days—much longer than any closing argument needs to be. I have long believed that lawyers should be able to make their key points and summarize their arguments in an hour or two. If it takes much longer, then I believe the lawyer has lost control of the case. In law school, lawyers learn that the attorneys have 100 percent attention of all twelve jurors for maybe ten or fifteen minutes.

After less than four hours of deliberations, the jury on October 2 found O. J. Simpson not guilty of the two counts of first-degree murder.

Even as the criminal trial was underway, the families of Nicole Brown Simpson and Ronald Goldman filed wrongful-death lawsuits against Simpson, accusing him of being liable for the deaths. The allegations in the lawsuits were nearly identical to the indictments charging Simpson with the murders. The civil complaint sought an undisclosed amount of money for damages.

Civil murder cases are few and far between. Most victims of crimes are satisfied to rely on the criminal justice system to hold alleged perpetrators of criminal activity accountable for their actions. But every once in a while, victims' families hire their own private lawyers and sue suspected criminals. It usually happens in cases where prosecutors have decided against charging the defendant with a crime or where the families feel the criminal courts went soft on the criminal defendant.

Under the law, it is not double jeopardy to pursue both civil and criminal charges against a defendant for the same offense. It would be double jeopardy only if prosecutors tried to put Simpson on trial a second time after the first jury found him not guilty. The civil case did not involve state prosecutors. In addition, civil lawsuits cannot impose prison sentences, only financial damages. Civil juries don't find people guilty; they declare defendants "liable."

One of the better-known examples of crime victims suing after being dissatisfied with the criminal prosecution is the case of New York subway shooter Bernard Goetz. After a criminal jury acquitted Goetz of attempted murder charges for shooting three youths on a subway in 1984, one of the victims, Darrell Cabey, filed a civil lawsuit. Confined to a wheelchair and suffering permanent brain damage, Cabey charged Goetz with reckless and outrageous conduct. The civil jury agreed and awarded Cabey $43 million in damages.

Normally, criminal defendants are not good targets for civil murder lawsuits because suspected killers are not wealthy. Cabey, for example, never collected the $43 million because Goetz's annual salary was a mere $20,000. So as a result, there is seldom money to get from the defendant even if the victims' families win in court. Not so with O. J. Simpson, who was worth a reported $10 million. When Simpson was acquitted by the criminal jury, Fred Goldman, Ron's father, swore he would never quit in his pursuit of justice.

The civil trial started on October 23, 1996, and lasted just three months. The jury heard 101 witnesses. On February 4, 1997, the jury found for the plaintiffs and awarded the victims' families $8.5 million in compensatory or actual damages. One week later, the same jury ordered Simpson to pay an additional $25 million in punitive damages. Lawyers for Simpson are still appealing the verdict.

There were several significant differences between the criminal and civil trials that explain the different verdicts. First, Goldman filed the complaint in Santa Monica, where they were sure to get a more favorable jury pool. Indeed, the civil jury consisted of nine white people, one black person, one Hispanic person, and one Asian person. Second, the plaintiffs' lawyers did a much better job of presenting the evidence against Simpson in a quicker, more effective manner. They avoided the pitfalls that befell prosecutors, including the Mark Fuhrman fiasco. Third, O. J. Simpson was required in the civil trial to answer critical and devastating questions under oath— questions he avoided in the criminal case by deciding not to testify. In criminal trials, defendants have a Fifth Amendment right against self-incrimination. There is no such protection in civil cases, because a defendant's personal liberties are not at stake in civil trials.

Finally, it does not take as much evidence for juries in civil

219

trials to rule against defendants. In civil trials, plaintiffs have to prove a mere "preponderance of the evidence" to win. That's been interpreted as 51 percent. By contrast, jurors in criminal trials must find that prosecutors have proven their case "beyond a reasonable doubt," which is a significantly higher standard. So, jurors in the civil case could still have some doubts or even significant doubts about Simpson's guilt and still find him liable for the deaths.

That being said, the issues in the civil and criminal cases were essentially identical. Did O. J. kill Nicole Brown Simpson and Ronald Goldman? In both cases, the prosecutors and plaintiffs needed to prove the same three elements:

1. Simpson had motivation or reasons to kill them both.
2. Simpson had the opportunity or ability to kill them.
3. Evidence—either direct or circumstantial—links Simpson to the slayings.

Prosecutors and plaintiffs' lawyers had no trouble showing that O. J. had motive in the slayings. A number of witnesses testified in both the criminal and the civil trials that Simpson was an abusive husband and a jealous ex-husband who possessed an explosive temper—all surprising to most of us who were previously unaware of this side of the former star. Family and friends told jurors that Simpson had actually stalked Nicole since their divorce in 1992.

Denise Brown, Nicole's sister, testified that Simpson once picked her sister up and threw her against a wall because he was angry she wouldn't do as he told her. She said she saw Simpson the day of the slayings at the dance recital and that he was mad at Nicole even then. He looked "scary," she said, "like a mad man."

Ron Shipp, Simpson's friend, told the jury that O. J. had confided to him a few weeks earlier that Simpson had had "dreams of killing Nicole."

And there was the now-infamous New Year's Day episode in which Nicole called authorities to their Brentwood home. When police arrived, Nicole's eye was black and her lip was bleeding. She was standing outside their home in near hysterics.

"He's going to kill me," she yelled out.

Simpson, wearing a bathrobe, responded, "I don't want that woman sleeping in my bed anymore. I got two women and I don't want that woman in my bed anymore."

After calming down both individuals, the officers informed Simpson that his wife wanted to file domestic abuse charges against him. "This is a family matter," O. J. said. "Why do you want to make a big deal about it? We can handle it."

Throughout their marriage, Nicole called police eight times claiming he had hit her or that he was threatening to hit her. In some of the 911 calls, Nicole is heard begging for help. Her voice is filled with absolute terror.

Maybe the most devastating evidence regarding motive in the civil and criminal trials came from Nicole herself in her diary. She wrote that Simpson would slap or beat her while the couple had sex. The diary also confirmed that he was stalking her.

"O. J. is following me again, Mommy," she wrote. "I'm scared. I go to the gas station, he's there. I go to the Payless Shoe Store, he's there. I'm driving and he's behind me."

Jurors at both trials also saw a workout or exercise tape in which Simpson is seen doing aerobic-style exercises with ease. The tape had two effects. First, it undermined the defense's contention that Simpson's football career had left his body so physically battered that he did not have the mobility, agility, or strength to overpower these two younger, physically fit individuals. Second, the tape shows Simpson running in place. As he throws jabs in the air, Simpson says men can pretend that they are "working out with your wife, if you know what I mean."

221

The second key issue for both prosecutors and plaintiffs' lawyers was to prove that Simpson had time and opportunity to commit the slayings. To accomplish this, the attorneys had to show that Simpson was at or near the scene of the crime at the time the crime took place. It would be very difficult to win a murder case against Simpson if Simpson could prove that he was out of town when the crime occurred or was with friends at the time the murders took place.

This part of the case required the lawyers to establish the exact time the attacks occurred and the whereabouts of Simpson at the time of the murders. To do so, prosecutors in the criminal trial and plaintiffs' lawyers in the civil case used various eyewitness and forensic testimony to develop a timeline of the night in question.

Police knew from telephone records and from personal testimony that Nicole had called Ron Goldman regarding her mother's sunglasses about 9:45 P.M. Eyewitnesses told jurors in both trials that Goldman left the restaurant about 9:50 P.M.

At 9:40 P.M., Simpson and houseguest Brian "Kato" Kaelin returned home in O. J.'s Bentley from McDonald's. According to Kaelin, Simpson said he was going to his bedroom to shower and pack for a late-night flight to Chicago. Simpson told police he also had gone outside in his backyard to practice his golf swing. Phone records show that Simpson tried calling his girlfriend, Victoria's Secret model Paula Barbieri, on the cell phone in his car.

Limousine driver Allan Park arrived at Simpson's home at 10:25 P.M. to take him to the airport. Park said he waited in the car until 10:40 P.M., when he walked to the front door and rang the buzzer to the home's intercom system. But he did not get an answer.

Kaelin, who didn't recall hearing Park on the intercom system, said he heard three thumps on the wall outside his bedroom at about 10:45 P.M.

Park testified that at 10:55 P.M. he saw a large shadowy figure enter the home through the front door. Park said the shadow appeared to be that of a tall black man weighing about two hundred pounds. Five minutes later, Simpson responded on the intercom, saying he had fallen asleep and would be down in a minute. At 11:01 P.M., O. J. opened his front door and climbed in the limo. Park said that Simpson was carrying a small black bag. When the driver offered to put the bag in the trunk of the car, Simpson wouldn't let him touch the bag. There was never an explanation for what was in the bag or what happened to it. A skycap at LAX said he saw Simpson near a trash bin, although he said he never saw Simpson put anything in it.

It was also about 10:55 P.M. that Steven Schwab, Nicole's neighbor, spotted Nicole's Akita a few blocks away from her home. He said that the dog acted agitated.

At 11:30 P.M., Simpson boarded American Airlines flight 668 bound for Chicago. It departed on time at 11:45 P.M.

About midnight, two other neighbors were walking their dog when they came across the Akita. They decided to take him back home to Nicole. A few minutes later, they discovered the bodies. They saw the body of Nicole lying near the front of the gate of the condo, at the foot of the stairs that led to her front door. Her body was curled up in a fetal position. Just two yards away, they spotted the body of Ronald Goldman leaning up against a tree stump and an iron fence.

Police records show that the neighbors dialed 911 at 12:10 A.M.

This timeline leaves open a window for Simpson to have left Kato Kaelin at his home at 9:45 P.M., driven the few miles in the Bronco to Nicole's condo, committed the murders, and then driven home by 10:45 P.M. But that window is very small and very tight.

The key for prosecutors was establishing the time of death for Nicole and Ron at 10:15 P.M. But here's where the problem arises. In most homicide cases, the police call the medical examiner's office immediately to notify them that a murder has taken place. It is important for the medical examiner or the medical examiner's investigators to examine the body as quickly as possible to determine the time of death.

According to medical examiner records and courtroom testimony, Los Angeles police arrived at the crime scene about 12:15 A.M., but they did not notify the Los Angeles medical examiner that there was a murder until 6:30 A.M. Even at that time, the police did not ask the medical examiner to come to the crime scene—they only told a representative of the office to stand by for a possible call. At 8:15 A.M., police called the medical examiner, informing her of the homicides and giving her the address of the homicides. A few minutes later, an investigator for the medical examiner arrived at Nicole's condo. However, the investigator testified that she was prevented by police from examining the bodies until 10:30 A.M.

There are three methods by which forensic pathologists determine time of death. None alone is exact or precise. But when you take the three methods together, a pretty accurate estimate can be made.

The first way is by determining the temperature of the body. When someone dies, the body begins to lose its heat. This is called algor mortis. The cooler the body temperature, the longer the person has been deceased.

Another method is by judging the level of rigor mortis or the stiffening of the muscles of the dead person. When someone dies, his or her muscles naturally begin to tighten. The longer a person has been dead, the stiffer the muscles.

And third, there is the livor mortis examination. When a person dies, gravity causes blood to settle at the bottom of the body or the part of the body lowest to the ground. This is referred to medically as livor mortis. The more the blood has settled, the longer the person has been deceased.

These tests are more reliable the sooner that the medical examiner is able to assess the condition of the body. By not allowing the medical examiner's investigator to examine the body, any ability to accurately determine the time of death was botched. As a result, the best estimate of time of death listed by the medical examiner was somewhere between 9 P.M. and midnight—a completely useless estimate.

This finding certainly allowed prosecutors and plaintiffs' lawyers to contend that the murders could have occurred at 10:15 P.M. to meet their tight timeline. However, the official estimate also opened the door for defense attorneys to argue that the deaths just as likely could have occurred at 11 P.M., which was after Simpson had been picked up by his limo driver. If the medical examiner had been able to examine the bodies right away to determine the time of death, it might have eliminated one of Simpson's defenses. Instead, because of this major misstep, the Los Angeles police actually strengthened Simpson's defense.

There were a series of mistakes or missteps by the police and medical examiners that led to Simpson's acquittal in the criminal trial. This was the first of those major blunders.

However, it is good to remember that the evidence about Simpson's temper and spousal abuse, as well as the testimony regarding Simpson's whereabouts at the time of the slayings, were just circumstantial evidence. While circumstantial evidence is still evidence, it is not as strong or reliable as direct physical or scientific evidence.

Direct evidence is evidence that directly connects Simpson to the crime scene and the homicides. It is the most damning kind of evidence against a criminal defendant. When Los Angeles prosecutors walked into court against Simpson, they were loaded with direct evidence. Not only did authorities have a lot of direct evidence, but it also appeared to be overwhelming evidence of O. J.'s guilt. As a former prosecutor and now as a medical examiner who most frequently testifies for the state, I dreamed about having cases with this much direct physical and forensic evidence against a defendant. "The physical evidence putting O. J. Simpson at the crime scene at the time these murders occurred is staggering," Assistant District Attorney Marcia Clark told jurors. "The evidence leaves no doubt."

The strength of the state's case started with the autopsies. Unfortunately for the authorities, it's also where their case started to unravel. Trial lawyer F. Lee Bailey sent me forty pages of police investigative materials, including the autopsy reports. The autopsy reported four stab wounds to Nicole Simpson's neck, three stab wounds to the scalp, two cuts on the right hand, and one cut on the left hand. "Death is attributable to multiple sharp force injuries, including a deep incised wound of the neck and multiple stab wounds to the neck," the autopsy stated. "The sharp force injuries led to the transection of the left and right arteries, and the incisions of the left and right internal jugular veins causing fatal exsanguinating hemorrhage."

The wound to the neck was five inches long and two inches deep. The edges of the wound were smooth, indicating it was not a serrated knife that had been used in the attacks. The wounds on the hands were defense wounds, as she held up her hands to protect the rest of her body from the brutal knife attack. The neck wounds were so deep that her head was barely connected to her body. The toxicology report found no evidence of illegal drugs in her blood and a blood-alcohol level of only 0.02 percent, which is equivalent to two glasses of wine.

Ronald Lyle Goldman's autopsy showed he suffered more than two dozen stab wounds to the face, neck, scalp, chest, abdomen, thighs, and hands. The fatal injury was a three-inch-long stab wound to the left side of the neck, which severed the jugular vein. The toxicology tests found no evidence of alcohol or illegal drugs in Goldman's body.

As I sifted through the reports Bailey had sent me, one suddenly jumped out. It was the minutes of an internal meeting conducted by the Los Angeles County coroner's official in the days immediately following the murders and the autopsies. As I reviewed the document, I counted no fewer than thirty errors committed during the autopsies— errors that the medical examiner's staff admitted to in the meeting.

For example, a bottle of liver bile was improperly marked as urine. The two bodies were kept overnight in unlocked and unsecured crypts, providing access to anyone wishing to tamper with them. Nicole's stomach contents were accidentally discarded. By examining how much food, the condition of the food in the stomach, and how much of it had been digested, forensic scientists could have helped determine time of death. Nicole's body was never examined for sexual assault. And most important, the medical examiners did not properly examine the stab wounds to see if the wounds could have been inflicted by a fifteen-inch knife, as prosecutors contended.

These errors were inexcusable. Combined, this was the second major snafu in the state's case. Not only did these significant missteps open the door for the defense to portray the medical examiners as the Keystone Cops, but they also opened the door to allegations of evidence tampering.

Los Angeles County coroner Lakshmanan Sathyavagiswaran admitted to the jury under oath that his office had made between thirty and forty errors in handling the evidence. The biggest problem, he said, was that his office was not called to examine the bodies for such a long time. As a result, he continued, the best estimate he could make regarding time of death was between 9 P.M. and 12:45 A.M. Otherwise, Dr. Sathyavagiswaran defended the basic findings of his office as accurate. Using graphic photographs of the bodies and the crime scene, he recreated the attacks for jurors.

The assailant began his terror by stabbing Nicole in the neck four times as she stood outside her condo. He then knocked her unconscious by ramming her head into the steel gate that surrounded her complex, according to Dr. Sathyavagiswaran. That is when Ron Goldman showed up. The attacker surprised Goldman by grabbing him from behind, forcing him into a small gated area that was smaller than six feet by four feet. Dr. Sathyavagiswaran testified that the assailant slashed Goldman's neck twice.

"If Mr. Goldman was confronted by the assailant in this confined area, he has no means to escape," he said. "He has no place to escape. He's stuck there. He was held so he couldn't move, so these controlled cuts could be made."

While Goldman received several other knife wounds, it was these two to the neck that were fatal, Dr. Sathyavagiswaran told the jury. As Goldman lay bleeding to death, the attacker stabbed him in the right chest. The knife went through the seventh rib and the right lung.

At this point, Dr. Sathyavagiswaran testified, the assailant turned his anger once again to Nicole, who he said was probably unconscious at the time. He said the attacker used his left hand to grab the victim's head by her hair and placed his foot on Nicole's back. The assailant pulled her head up, exposing her throat. The knife in his right hand, the attacker then slit her throat so deeply he almost decapitated her.

"I would say she died within a few minutes, probably much less than a minute," he said. "She would have gone into rapid shock with this massive injury. I felt that the injuries sustained could have been in rapid succession."

Dr. Sathyavagiswaran told jurors that the entire attack, from beginning to end, lasted only a minute. "A minute is a long time," he said. "I mean, we all heat our coffee cups in the microwave oven, and you know, it takes a long time. You take any knife and just go home and plunge it quickly and you'll see you can do fifteen thrusts in about fifteen seconds. It doesn't take that long to do a sharp-force injury with a sharp knife."

Although the recreation of the night of the crime was extremely well presented and very effective, I have big problems with his interpretation of the injuries, crime scene photographs, and the autopsies. To me, the scenario he offers simply doesn't match what I believe the evidence shows us. This is not to attack Dr. Sathyavagiswaran personally or his abilities as a forensic pathologist. Instead, I have a different opinion about what circumstances would produce this evidence.

Remember, these were stabbings, not shootings. Stabbings are not nearly as clean or precise as shootings. Stabbings are more dynamic because people are moving, trying to get away, or trying to fight back. In this case especially, Nicole and Ron were young, athletic, vivacious individuals. Neither of them was on drugs or under the influence of much alcohol. They certainly didn't stand still to allow the wounds to be inflicted unchallenged. However, the state's scenario of the crime scene allowed no room for any attempt by either victim to try to get away.

Proof of their flawed argument can be found in the lack of blood found at the crime scene. Both of these victims had their carotid arteries and jugular veins slashed. The blood from each must have spurted several feet into the air. In addition, the victims were under attack, causing tremendous fear, which would have resulted in their blood pressures skyrocketing. That would have significantly increased the force with which blood coursed through their aortas.

Keep in mind, blood is much thicker than water. It doesn't just seep into the ground undetected. When blood dries, it sticks or gels on skin or clothes or wherever it settles, and it is very difficult to clean up quickly and thoroughly.

With these kinds of stab wounds, blood should have been everywhere. The attacker must have been soaked in blood. The blood must have squirted all over the clothes and body of the assailant. Yet the police discovered very little blood anywhere except on the clothes of the victims. If Simpson was the killer, he

229

must have been covered in blood when he left the crime scene. And he would almost assuredly have transferred significant portions of it to his vehicle, to the white carpet in his house, to other clothes, and so on. Yet police found very little blood from the victims anywhere. This should have given the authorities great pause in developing their theory about what happened.

During his testimony, Dr. Michael Baden testified that the blood spatter patterns at the crime scene were inconsistent with the state's theory. He said that the bloodstains on the cement near Nicole's body make it appear as if she were about eighteen inches off the ground when the final, fatal cutting of the throat took place. He also said that he found bruises on Ron Goldman's knuckles, indicating that he must have struck the attacker. That also blew holes in the prosecution's scenario about how it happened.

The physical evidence that could and should have been most damaging to Simpson was the bloodstains found on his Bronco, on a glove found near his house, and on a pair of socks. In addition, there was the blood of a third person found near the crime scene. Blood evidence can be devastating because it can prove, through DNA testing, that a person was at the scene of the crime. A single drop of blood may seem insignificant, but because of today's technology, it can be the exclusive evidence that sends someone to prison.

The first key piece of evidence, tested by the California Department of Justice laboratory and by Cellmark Diagnostics, was a right-handed glove discovered outside of Simpson's guesthouse. Authorities found blood on the glove's middle finger. Testing proved that the blood was a mixture of Nicole's blood and Ron's blood. This was extremely crucial evidence against Simpson.

The two socks found at the foot of Simpson's bed were the second key physical blood evidence. DNA testing found that blood splatters on each sock came from Nicole. Dr. Robin Cotton, director of Cellmark, told jurors that the chances that the blood on

230

the socks came from an individual other than Nicole were an astronomical 9.7 billion to one. When one realizes that there are only about 6 billion people on the planet, this was extremely explosive evidence against Simpson.

The droplets of blood in the Bronco turned out to be Simpson's. Prosecutors claimed he had cut himself at the crime scene. The defense attributed the cuts to an injury he had sustained earlier that same day—cuts he had told police about in their interview with him the day after the slayings. To support this, defense lawyers called three witnesses. The first was a graduate student at UCLA who sat next to Simpson on the airplane. He said that he had looked at Simpson's hands to see if O. J. had a Super Bowl ring. In doing so, he said he got a good look at Simpson's hands and he saw no evidence of fresh cuts. The next two witnesses were employees of Hertz, who said they didn't notice fresh cuts when Simpson arrived in Chicago the night of the slayings, but did notice fresh cuts the next morning, when they took him back to the airport to fly home. Simpson's lawyers argued that this supported his contention that he obtained the cuts when he broke a glass in his hotel room when he had heard that Nicole had been murdered.

And finally, five drops of blood discovered at the scene of the crime matched Simpson's DNA. The state's DNA expert testified that there were 170 million to one odds against the blood coming from someone other than Simpson.

DNA fingerprinting is essentially a lock. DNA testing and matches have been challenged in courts all around the world, and uniformly judges have said it is valid science. Most important, it cannot produce false positives. In other words, there is no chance whatsoever that a DNA test is going to come back positively identifying the defendant when it is not the defendant's blood or body tissue. Tainted or contaminated blood will not result in a false positive, unless it is contaminated with the defendant's own blood.

Deoxyribonucleic acid (DNA) is a substance within a person's blood, skin, hair, or other body tissues and fluids that contains an individual's genetic blueprint. Using samples of these, scientists can map genetic patterns. Just like fingerprints, DNA is exclusive to a particular person. DNA is made up of four basic chemical bases: adenine, guanine, thymine, and cytosine. Like the letters in the alphabet, each chemical base in DNA helps establish a genetic pattern.

The key method in testing DNA at the time was restriction fragment length polymorphism, or RFLP. The RFLP tests take up to six weeks to complete, but their accuracy is unbelievable. Using scientific databases, crime lab experts can narrow a DNA pattern to one in a million people or even one in a billion people, which is essentially a match.

The RFLP is a seven-step test. First, scientists obtain DNA from blood or other body tissues. Second, each DNA sample is chemically divided into fragments using restriction enzymes. Third, the DNA samples are placed in a gel. An electric current running through the gel separates the DNA samples into bands. In the fourth step, the bands, which are visible at this stage, are transferred to nylon membranes. Step five requires that the radioactive DNA probes be applied to the membranes and bind to matching DNA sequences. X-ray film is placed next to the membranes in stage six. The film, once it is developed, reveals a pattern of bands where the radioactive probes bind to the DNA fragments. This DNA profile is the genetic fingerprint. The final DNA fingerprints are patterns of light and dark bands that look similar to bar codes. In the seventh and final step, scientists compare their samples for a match.

Because of the strength and validity of DNA evidence, the defense had only one route it could take: to argue that the evidence was planted and that O. J. was being framed for the slayings. This defense is tried many times every year in courts all across the country. It seldom works, because most of the time it's not true. But the Simpson case had proven to be an anomaly in every other respect, and it would do so again.

Defense lawyers learned that some of the blood Simpson had voluntarily allowed police to take from him was missing. According to the nurse who took Simpson's blood, he withdrew 8 cubic centimeters (cc) of blood. But when the vials of blood were turned into the crime lab for testing, there were only 6.5 cc of blood. About 1.5 cc—the equivalent of thirty drops of blood—were missing. The vials were in police custody for several hours between the time that the nurse took Simpson's blood and the time it was logged at the crime lab.

The claim that the blood had been planted on the socks gained steam when Dr. Fredric Rieders, the forensic toxicologist, told jurors that he, too, had tested the bloodstains on the socks. Yes, it was definitely a match with Simpson, but, he said, he also found something else in the blood on the socks—a chemical called ethyl-enediaminetetraacetic acid. EDTA, as it is more commonly referred to, is a chemical preservative chemists add to blood to store it for testing. EDTA is not naturally found in blood.

There is only one explanation for this: blood previously taken from Simpson and preserved was placed on the socks.

Then came two more revelations about the socks. Drs. Baden and Lee examined the state's physical evidence very soon after Simpson's arrest. Both had examined the socks, and both say they saw no bloodstains on either sock. Prosecutors admit that the police didn't notice or report the bloodstains on the socks until six weeks later.

The second development occurred during the testimony of Herb MacDonell, a nationally renowned bloodstain expert and criminalist. His opinion was that the blood on the socks had not gotten there via a natural blood spatter. Instead, the blood had been applied to the socks through "direct compression." In other words, someone intentionally put the blood on the socks. He pointed out that the bloodstain was identical on both sides of the sock. The only way for that to happen, he said, is if there was not a foot in the sock at the time the blood was applied. This completely supported the defense's contention that the blood evidence had been planted.

But that still left the glove with Nicole and Ron's blood on it. The glove had been found by Los Angeles police detective Mark Fuhrman. Prosecutors at first trumpeted Fuhrman as a hero cop whose solid police work had unearthed the key evidence against Simpson. Rumors abounded that Fuhrman was a racist or had used racial slurs in the past. Defense attorney Bailey tried to cross-examine the detective about his use of racial slurs, which he adamantly denied. In fact, he said he hadn't used the "N" word in more than ten years. Prosecutors frequently came to Fuhrman's defense, calling him a good and trusted police officer.

Weeks later, the defense stumbled on a series of startling revelations. First, two women who had dated Fuhrman came forward separately to say the officer had used racial slurs in their presence. Both testified that Fuhrman told them he hated interracial couples and that he used his position as a police officer to physically abuse black people and to plant evidence against them.

The witness who sealed Fuhrman's fate and devastated the state's case was Laura Hart McKinney, a North Carolina college professor who had been interviewing Fuhrman about life on a police force for a movie script she was writing. The interviews had been tape-recorded. McKinney didn't want to turn the taped interviews over to defense lawyers for Simpson. Only after a judge ordered her to give them the tapes did she comply.

On the witness stand, McKinney said Fuhrman had used the "N" word during their interviews forty-two times. Several of those times, she said, had occurred in interviews since Simpson's arrest.

Subpoenaed by defense attorneys to retake the witness stand, Fuhrman repeatedly refused to testify, citing his Fifth Amendment right under the U.S. Constitution not to incriminate himself in a crime. The implication was clear: the glove, the socks, and other evidence was probably planted against Simpson. As a result, the state's entire case was contaminated. F. Lee Bailey's cross-examination of Fuhrman regarding the use of the "N" word was one of the most brilliant and devastating examples in the annals of courtroom tactics on how to succinctly dissect a witness who is not telling the truth.

The state's case took one more blow. Dr. Lee during his testimony told jurors that he had found "imprints" on the sidewalk and on Ron Goldman's blue jeans. The imprints, he said, were probably shoe prints because they were all identical. He said the shoe print was not the same as the size twelve Bruno Magli shoe that FBI agents identified at the crime scene. Authorities pointed out to jurors that Simpson wore a size twelve, though they never found Bruno Magli shoes.

The prosecution's once incredibly strong case had fallen apart. For many, the trial had somehow gone from Simpson as the bad guy to the Los Angeles police as the bad guys. Legal experts, who once described the state's case as a slam-dunk, now agreed that Simpson would probably walk free.

And he did.

On October 3, 1995, at 1 P.M. EST, with all the networks interrupting their regular broadcasts, the jury in the criminal case reported their findings.

"We, the jury, in the above titled action, find the defendant, Orenthal James Simpson, not guilty of the crime of murder." Seconds later, they repeated it another time.

By contrast, the jury in the civil case on February 4, 1997, found Simpson "liable" for the two deaths. They awarded the families $8.5 million in actual or compensatory damages and $25 million in punitive damages.

"We came to the conclusion that Mr. Simpson should not profit from these murders," juror Stephen Strati said.[1]

Added fellow juror Orville Bigelow, "He was a hero to us, and he betrayed us all. He's a charming man and a nice man, but charming men kill. There's just no way anyone could have planted all that evidence."[2]

Seven weeks after the civil trial ended, Simpson auctioned off his Brentwood home and turned over many of his valuables and assets to court officials to help meet the judgment against him. Among the valuables Simpson turned over to the court were his 1968 Heisman Trophy, a $25,000 Andy Warhol painting, a $40,000 gold necklace with eighty-nine diamonds, a $26,000 fur coat, and many of his golf clubs. California law does not allow courts to touch or seize the $25,000 a month Simpson receives from his football pension fund.

After the trial, Fred Goldman told reporters he would forfeit his right to collect all the money against Simpson if O. J. would publicly confess to the homicides. But Simpson immediately rejected the offer.

The civil trial included no *new* evidence, with one exception: Simpson was forced to give a full deposition under oath to the plaintiffs' lawyers. And he didn't fare well, though he always proclaimed his innocence. Jurors in the civil case got to see Simpson squirm when confronted with overwhelming documentation of spousal abuse.

Beyond that, the two trials featured essentially the same evidence. But the plaintiffs' lawyers did a much better job of presenting it than the state prosecutors. They avoided calling Detective Fuhrman to the witness stand, thereby taking a big bite out of the defense's claim of police frame-up. And the plaintiffs' attorneys were helped by the fact that their trial was in wealthy Santa Monica, where a great majority of the jurors were white, women, and very conservative. In addition, Judge Hiroshi Fujisaki, who handled the civil trial, ruled with an iron fist.

What I believe happened in this case is simple: the police firmly believed O. J. was the culprit. However, they didn't have enough evidence, especially solid physical evidence, connecting Simpson to the crime scene. So, I believe some members of the police decided to enhance or even fabricate evidence against Simpson. These police officers saw it as a way to firm up a case against a man they were convinced was guilty.

This goes completely against what our Founding Fathers believed. It's directly opposed to our system of justice and our sense of fairness. Former Supreme Court justice Oliver Wendell Holmes once wrote that it is much better to set a thousand guilty men free than to falsely convict one innocent man.

Here's a better way of understanding why we cannot allow police to fabricate evidence against criminal defendants: If you can railroad a guilty man to prison, you can railroad an innocent man to prison, too.

So, what really did happen in this case?

Like most Americans, I believe O. J. probably was involved in the slayings, but I don't think he did it alone. He must have had help. And it could be that Simpson was not the person wielding the knife. The physical evidence—the multiple footprints at the crime scene, the lack of blood at the crime scene, the forcefulness with which the crimes were committed, the time restraints during which the crimes were committed—strongly supports the theory that there was a second attacker involved.

That's why I believe that both juries were correct. The plaintiffs' lawyers clearly convinced the civil jury that a preponderance of the evidence shows that Simpson was responsible for the slayings. In my opinion, the evidence strongly supports that verdict.

By contrast, the state simply didn't prove beyond a reasonable doubt its claim that Simpson committed these crimes alone. Their theory of Simpson as the lone attacker had many holes. And the authorities ended up with dirty hands. Beyond a reasonable doubt is, as our Founding Fathers intended, a very high burden to overcome.

Chapter Eight

ROBERT BERDELLA

Madman or Just Murderer?

BEFORE JEFFREY DAHMER, there was Robert Berdella.

Both men were sex fiends and serial killers of the first order. Each lured young men, many of them drug-addicted or homeless, into their respective lairs. There, they slipped mind-numbing drugs into their food and drink that caused their prey to fall into a state of insensibility. The two repeatedly raped and tortured their victims. As if proud of their conquests, the pair documented their individual actions by taking photographs. And when the life had fled the physically and psychologically battered bodies of the victims, Berdella and Dahmer carved their kill into small pieces with saws and knives.

Berdella, like Dahmer, grew up in the Midwest. That such horrible acts could take place in the heartland of America seemed to shock people. Though there is no evidence that the two men ever met or even knew of each other, the similarities between them and their activities is remarkable. Both men confessed to their crimes. They were each sentenced to serve the rest of their life in prison. And both died behind bars a short time after they were convicted.

While the issue of guilt or innocence was never in question in either situation, the Berdella case offered an intriguing medical-legal question that Dahmer's did not: did Robert Berdella truly *intend* to kill his victims?

I was asked to become involved in the Berdella case in July 1992 by civil plaintiff's lawyers from Kansas City, Missouri. The attorneys represented the family of Todd Stoops, a homicide victim in the Berdella case. The family sued Berdella's estate and his insurance company, with which he had homeowner's protection, for the wrongful death of Stoops.

By the time I was consulted in the case, Berdella had already confessed to killing six young men, including Todd Stoops. He had pleaded guilty and was serving a life sentence. The criminal case was over.

Despite the horrific details of the case, I admitted to the trial lawyers who contacted me that I was completely unfamiliar with the Berdella case. That such a bizarre and distressing case slipped by me was surprising, since I read the *New York Times* and the Pittsburgh newspapers every day.

By contrast, Jeffrey Dahmer was in the newspaper on a daily basis following his arrest in September 1991 in Milwaukee, Wisconsin, for killing seventeen young men. The facts of the two cases were amazingly similar. I could not then, and cannot today, understand why the Berdella case did not attract as much news media interest as did Jeffrey Dahmer, especially since the Berdella case came to light more than three years prior to Dahmer.

It could be that Dahmer killed three times as many men.

Another important difference in the two cases is that Dahmer was a cannibal, a taboo that probably disgusts society even more than incest or bestiality. While Dahmer enjoyed his victims in the bedroom *and* kitchen, Berdella simply used his prey as sex toys that he could dominate, then discard without the notice of authorities.

But I believe that the single most significant reason that Robert Berdella did not receive as much publicity as Dahmer is because there was no criminal trial. The Dahmer trial was broadcast live from the courtroom to millions of television sets. Berdella, on the other hand, cut a deal with prosecutors in which he pleaded guilty to his crimes and gave a full confession. In exchange, the district attorney agreed not to seek the death penalty.

Consequently, the dramatic testimony was unveiled in a secret conference room in the basement of the Kansas City jail instead of in open court in front of a jury, television cameras, and newspaper reporters. There was no suspense-filled moment, as in the cases of Dahmer or O. J. Simpson, when the world awaited the jury's verdict of guilt or acquittal.

While Berdella's culpability or the cause of the six victims' deaths was never in doubt, the case offered two factors that forensic scientists, law enforcement officers, and lawyers seldom face. First, none of his victims' bodies were ever found. All we had to go on was his confession; a diary he kept in which he detailed the capture, abuse, and deaths of his victims; the photographs he took of them; and a couple of skulls discovered around his house. As a result, there were no autopsies for us to do, no medical tests to conduct, and very few forensic experiments to perform. Obviously, this was a very frustrating situation for a scientist.

The second fascinating aspect of this case was the brainchild of a very smart and innovative trial lawyer. In telephone conversations with the attorneys who represented Betty Ann Haste, who was Todd Stoops's mother, I learned that they had sued Berdella's estate and the insurance company that held the homeowners policy on Berdella's house. The lawsuit sought a whopping $1 billion in damages from Berdella's estate. The wrongful-death trial lasted less than two days. Berdella did not testify. From the beginning of the trial, plaintiff's lawyers told the Jackson County, Missouri, jury that they needed to send a message to Berdella and other would-be serial killers.

"You can award ten times all the money in the world," attorney John Turner told jurors in closing arguments, "and it wouldn't be enough money to compensate Stoops and his family for the torture he suffered at Berdella's hands. Your verdict needs to let him know what this jury said when they heard about this concentration camp behavior."[1]

Because Berdella had already confessed and pleaded guilty to the crimes, there were very few evidentiary surprises. The lawyers defending Berdella's estate basically offered no defense. What could they say? How could they defend his actions? What argument could they give that Todd Stoops's family did not deserve a large sum of money or that Robert Berdella should not be required to pay a large judgment?

But $1 billion? Even the plaintiff's lawyers admitted that they were aiming high. If the jury awarded them a tenth of that, or a mere $100 million, they would be satisfied.

The jurors took longer to pick a jury foreman than they did to agree that Berdella was liable for Todd Stoops's death. The touchy question was how much. The jury foreman initially put on the table for discussion the $1 billion figure that the plaintiff's lawyers had suggested to them. The first vote was eight to four in favor of awarding $1 billion. But in Missouri, nine of twelve jurors must agree in a civil case before a verdict is final. So the jurors each told what they thought an appropriate verdict would be. Their final choice stunned the courtroom and legal experts: $5 billion.

The National Center for State Courts, which oversees the operation of the state court systems, and the Administrative Office of the U.S. Courts, which does the same thing for the federal courts, both declared the judgment the largest jury award ever handed down in a wrongful-death or personal-injury lawsuit in the United States. The jury decided to give Stoops's family $2.5 billion for Todd's death and $2.5 billion for aggravating circumstances, which is the equivalent to punitive damages in other jurisdictions. After the trial, the jurors made known their disgust for Robert Berdella and his actions to news reporters.

"I felt like I was in the presence of evil, even though Berdella wasn't there," the jury foreman told the *Kansas City Star* on January 9, 1992. "We wanted to make a statement that there is no dollar-amount value on a human life."

"He didn't have any remorse or feelings," another juror told reporter Tom Jackman for an article he wrote about the verdict. "As we speak now, there are animals out there. This kind of thing makes the community aware."

While the plaintiff's lawyers were thrilled by the verdict, they knew this was the easy part of their case. Collecting the money was a different matter. Obviously, Berdella didn't have $5 billion. A trustee of his estate testified that Berdella had $8,000 in cash, which was the result of selling all of his belongings, and $55,000 in a trust fund from selling his house. In addition, Berdella worked in the state penitentiary's inmate labor program, earning $76 a month. At that rate, Berdella would be able to pay off the judgment in about 5.5 million years, excluding any interest.

With these excessive dollar amounts, it was obvious that the target of the lawyers was the deep pockets of Economy Fire and Casualty. But there was a problem with making the insurance company pay up. The liability insurance policy covered only accidental deaths.

How could anyone argue that the death of Todd Stoops or any of Berdella's victims were accidental? After all, he did kill them.

By its very definition, murder cannot be accidental. It was at this stage that lawyers for the Stoops family contacted me. They promised that I would be surprised at the evidence. The attorneys asked me to thoroughly review all the case files and then give my expert medical opinion on four simple issues:

1. Based on the available data, identify the cause of Todd Stoops's death.
2. Identify the conduct of Berdella that caused or directly contributed to cause Todd Stoops's death.
3. Explain the nature and severity of the injury Berdella caused when he "fisted" Todd Stoops.
4. Was the medical attention Berdella gave Stoops adequate to treat Todd's injury?
5. Did Berdella try to keep Stoops alive?

The medical-legal issues in question fascinated me, as did the facts in the case itself. I quickly agreed to join the plaintiff's legal team. A few days later, I received a large package in the mail with pounds of information designed to bring me up to date on the details of the case and the specific legal and medical controversies. The packet included:

1. several police investigative reports,
2. two dozen newspaper clips of the case,
3. a copy of the insurance policy,
4. copies of eighty-one graphic Polaroid photographs of the victims purportedly taken by Berdella and found by police in his home,
5. a copy of the 58-page diary Berdella kept on the capture, torture, and death of Stoops and five other young men, and
6. a three-volume, 717-page statement or confession by Berdella to prosecutors under oath.

The confession was by far the centerpiece evidence in the case. In the interview, Berdella gave authorities a quick history of his entire life. He told them how he met each of the young men, and he described for them in graphic detail how he persecuted his victims, how he watched each of them die, and how he disposed of their bodies. The story he told was certainly one of the most horrendous that I have heard in four decades of investigating homicides and other mysterious deaths.

Robert Berdella was born to Robert Andrew Berdella Sr. and Mary Berdella in Canton, Ohio, on January 31, 1949. The elder Berdella was a die-setter at a Ford Motor Company plant. Mrs. Berdella was a homemaker. When young Bobby was five, his family moved to Cuyahoga Falls, Ohio. He received A's in school and loved math, history, music, and art. In 1966 and 1967, he was a member of the National Honor Society. In high school, he participated in the stamp and algebra clubs. On weekends, he worked for the city's civic art center and public parks department helping art students set up their displays.

In 1965, Berdella's father died of a heart attack at the age of thirty-nine. Friends of the family told detectives that young Bobby, who was only sixteen at the time, was devastated by his dad's death. The summer he graduated from high school, his mother remarried and they moved to Berberton, Ohio.

Neither of his parents was very religious. His father was Roman Catholic and his mother was Presbyterian. Young Bobby was christened Catholic. However, he stopped attending church after his father died. Berdella later told psychologists that he became aware of his homosexual tendencies when he was an adolescent. He also said that when he was a teenager, he was raped by a man he worked for at a restaurant.

As an adult, Berdella stood 6 feet 2 inches, weighed about 180–190 pounds, had short, dark brown hair, and wore very thick glasses to correct his nearsightedness. Most people described him as a loner, someone who seldom spoke up in conversations. He wore conservative clothes—never shorts—and had a speech impediment. Because he hated the brightness of the sunlight, his skin remained pale white and never tanned. He also suffered from high blood pressure and hypertension, taking various medications for both. In high school, he expressed no interest in girls and started visiting gay bars.

Having turned eighteen and ready to leave home, Berdella moved to Kansas City in the fall of 1967 to attend the city's Art Institute. The school had given him a partial scholarship. He majored in painting and minored in ceramics and art history. He dreamed of becoming a college art professor. Needing some extra cash, he started working as a short-order cook in various restaurants across the city. Eventually, he moved up to more upscale and expensive restaurants and started developing a reputation as one of Kansas City's better, more experimental chefs. In fact, Berdella was such a good cook that the city's top country clubs started outbidding each other for his services. His specialties included lamb and veal prepared in a variety of ways.

After two and a half years, he became disillusioned with college and dropped out. "I very quickly found out I could make twice as much money flipping hamburgers as I could as a college professor," Berdella told prosecutors and detectives during his three-day confession.

Berdella became a poster boy for the hippie movement, complete with shoulder-length dark hair and a shaggy beard. Once an introvert, he was no longer shy about sharing his antigovernment and anti–family values opinions.

While Berdella was never known as a significant drug user, he did have a friend who supplied with him marijuana and various pills at cheap rates. Berdella would then sell the dope to his friends, making a little profit for himself. But during his junior year in college, he was arrested for selling amphetamines to a federal undercover agent. He agreed to plead guilty and was given a five-year suspended sentence. Less than a month later, he and some other students were arrested again for allegedly possessing marijuana and LSD. However, after spending five days in jail, the charges were dropped by police due to a lack of evidence.

In 1969, Berdella became tired of paying $175 a month in rent and started house shopping. He found the perfect spot at 4315 Charlotte Avenue. With only $100 down and a bright future as a chef, the bank gave him the loan and the Victorian-style, three-story wood-frame house was his. The house was in the middle-class community of Hyde Park, which sat on the edge of Kansas City's art district.

According to police reports, the spare bedroom in his new home soon became a storage facility for Berdella's newest interest: bizarre antiques and artifacts, many of which were Roman and Egyptian. Sometime in the mid-1970s, he decided to supplement his chef's income by trading and selling some of his artifacts. He developed business cards with his name, phone number, and his home address. The business cards also featured the words "Dragon nagari" and a dragon logo, which he discovered in a book on ancient legends called *The Illustrated History of Magic*. The symbol would later lead some police detectives to believe that Berdella was involved in some form of Satanic worship or the occult.

Throughout the seventies and early eighties, Robert Berdella's world flourished. His career as an accomplished chef at several of the more prominent Kansas City restaurants and country clubs gave him a distinguished status in the community. At the same time, his side business of buying, selling, and trading antiques and artifacts outgrew his home. Needing to expand, he leased booth space at the Old Westport Flea Market. He called his shop Bob's Bizarre Bazaar. He expanded his contacts to traders in Europe and South America to complement his already solid business ties to dealers in the Middle East.

247

The more he became involved with his artifact business, the less he cared about being a chef. In 1980, Berdella decided he wanted to give Bob's Bizarre Bazaar his full-time attention. His knowledge of the artifacts he sold was impressive to those who shopped at his store. Once again, Berdella's life went through a transformation—this time from a sixties hippie rebel to an entrepreneur of the eighties.

In another ironic twist, Berdella helped organize the South Hyde Park Crime Watch program, and even became its president in 1981. Neighbors said he was always friendly and helpful, though a bit arrogant.

In the late seventies, Berdella began taking in boarders. Most were young men with drug problems who had troubles with the law. In return for room and food, the young men would do various chores around the house or at the shop. The neighbors, while a bit uncertain or nervous about having a steady influx of unstable characters constantly coming and going in their community, applauded Berdella for taking the time to help out these troubled youths.

By 1983, however, neighbors thought Berdella was going beyond eccentric. No longer did he wave at those who lived near him, nor did he even return smiles. Around his yard was spread wood for his fireplace, while his porch was packed with junk he had rejected from his artifact business. In fact, many who once enjoyed small talk with him about the weather now found him rude and uncaring.

Meanwhile, young men continued to come and go from the house with increasing frequency. Then came Berdella's first major confrontation with police. In the fall of 1985, Kansas City detectives were investigating the disappearances of Jerry Howell, a nineteen-year-old man who had vanished in July 1984, and James Ferris, a twenty-five-year-old man who was last seen in September 1985.

Police had found a witness named Todd Stoops who knew Howell and Ferris. Stoops and some unidentified police informants claimed that they had last seen both men with a guy named Robert

Berdella. In fact, Stoops told detectives that the word on the street was that Berdella had injected Howell with a "hot shot"—street slang for a hybrid tranquilizer. Stoops was a male prostitute, who told police that he and his wife had stayed at Berdella's house on a couple of different occasions in an effort to get back on their feet. The detectives gave Todd Stoops one piece of advice: never go back to that house, and stay far away from Robert Berdella. Unfortunately, it was counsel that he would ignore.

Investigators staked out Berdella's home, waiting for him to return. When he did, they confronted him at the front door. Berdella admitted he had seen Howell on the last day the young man was seen, but that he had dropped him off at a nearby 7-Eleven convenience store. He adamantly denied any foul play.

Berdella also told police he knew Ferris. He said he allowed Ferris to stay at his house for a few days until he discovered that Ferris had stolen antiques from his home and had sold them to buy drugs. Again, Berdella denied giving Ferris any drugs or knowing what had happened to him.

Even so, the detectives were convinced that Berdella knew more than he was saying. For several weeks, they followed his every move. They would suddenly appear at his store, asking him questions and hounding him. But they had no evidence, so they reluctantly put away the case file, where it collected dust for the next couple of years.

The next time police came across Robert Berdella's name was April 2, 1988, at 10:28 A.M., the day before Easter. That's when a young man, his hands and arms bound by rope and bathrobe sashes, his mouth gagged by a washcloth and piano wire, jumped out of an open window in a two-story house to the ground. No one heard the thump of his body hitting the ground.

Completely naked, with the exception of a black spiked dog collar around his neck, Christopher Bryson stumbled across the street where he saw a water company meter man. Bryson appeared to be semiconscious. His face was pale, his body trembling, and he couldn't stop crying. In an extremely low voice, the young man asked the meter man to call the police.

Over the next hour, police and neighbors were horrified at the tale Chris Bryson told them. These are the details that he could remember: Berdella lured him into the house by offering to give him cocaine. Bryson thought Berdella was probably gay and that he wanted sex in return for the free drugs—a proposition Bryson was willing to accept. After a couple of beers, Berdella came up behind Bryson when he wasn't looking and hit him in the back of the skull with a twenty-inch iron pipe. Berdella carried Bryson's 5-foot, 10-inch, 160-pound frame upstairs to a bedroom. There he produced a syringe and needle and injected something directly into Bryson's neck. Within minutes, Bryson passed out.

When he awoke later, his hands and feet were tied to the bedposts. At first, Bryson resisted his attacker by turning away his head, trying to scream or fight. But there appeared to be no escape. Berdella punished each of Bryson's protests by gouging his eyes or sending electrical shocks through his body. Berdella attached electrodes to Bryson's genitals, and then powered up an electric transformer that sent 7,700 volts of electricity through his body. This lasted four days.

Bryson escaped when Berdella left the house the morning of April 2, 1988, to go to work. Some of the drugs had worn off, allowing Bryson to collect his thoughts and develop a plan for an escape. He called out Berdella's name, just to make sure he was gone. Bryson began wiggling his hands around until one of the ropes holding him to the bedpost came loose. But the ropes on his feet were too tight, and he simply didn't have the energy to release them. That's when he spotted a pack of matches Berdella had dropped on the floor. Using a handful of matches, Bryson eventually burned away the strands that bound him.

He thought about simply walking out the front door, but he feared that Berdella might be hiding downstairs or waiting for him on the porch. He walked to the window in the bedroom. To his surprise, it was not locked or nailed shut and opened easily. He tried lowering himself onto a ledge below, but he slipped and fell about eighteen feet to the ground.

With Chris Bryson's testimony, investigators had enough probable cause to obtain a search warrant and enter Berdella's home. Inside, detectives found hard-core pornographic magazines. They also found clips of newspaper articles featuring some of the nation's biggest serial killers and books on devil worshiping and the occult.

Their biggest discovery was packages of Polaroid photographs in one of Berdella's bedrooms that stunned detectives. They showed young men performing oral and anal sex with Berdella. Other photographs featured syringes and needles sticking out of the throats of young men. Most of the pictures showed naked men, their mouths gagged, handcuffed or tied with ropes to a bed. Many of them revealed Berdella apparently raping the victims with a cucumber. And the pictures showed Berdella attaching electrodes to the young men's genitals, just as Chris Bryson had claimed.

The young men in the photographs appeared either in a drug-induced, semiconscious state or with the unmistakable look of terror in their eyes. These pictures, combined with the earlier reports involving the two missing men, Jerry Howell and James Ferris, confirmed police suspicions that Robert Berdella was involved in heinous crimes.

On a small wooden nightstand in the room where Bryson claimed he had been tortured, detectives recovered what appeared to be a personal diary. Page after page was filled with dates, times, lists of sexual acts, use of drugs, and various responses. The lawyers sent me a copy of the personal journal to examine. The

251

diary appeared to detail Berdella's observations and actions. For example:

"Tuesday, 6/17/86, 4:20 P.M., bathtub, vomited in toilet."

"Wednesday, 6/18/86, 5:45 P.M., Chlorpromazine 6cc, buttocks, EKG to legs, back and arms. He attempted some resistance."

"Thursday, 6/19/86, 3:00 A.M., He was tied. Some whipping with a belt strap. Cucumber rape, sodomization. 'Please, don't hurt me.'"

This kind of description went on and on, but there were no names. It left investigators shaking their heads in disbelief, in utter disgust. Criminal psychologists say that sexual sadists frequently write down their actions in an effort to thoroughly document the things they are doing.

Crime scene experts walked through the house dusting for fingerprints. They collected the bed's sheets, pillowcases, and blankets, anything that might produce DNA, or hair or blood samples to identify possible victims. Every corner, every bookshelf, and every closet was packed full with items. Berdella was obviously a pack rat in the extreme.

Upstairs in Berdella's bedroom, detectives searched through his dresser drawers, sifting through clothes and shoes and boxes, when an officer who opened the bedroom closet door found himself staring nose-to-nose at a human skull. Next to it was a small envelope that contained a set of teeth.

After a quick private meeting at Berdella's home, detectives agreed they needed two things: dead bodies and Berdella. To this point, they had only Chris Bryson as a victim, lots of rumors, a few bizarre pieces of what could be evidence, and some very sickening photographs.

Their first step was the excavation of the backyard. With the help of a backhoe, they found dozens of animal bones and some glass jars filled with bird feathers. Then, on the third scoop, the detectives couldn't believe their eyes. There was a head with hair still attached and what appeared to be a vertebra.

"Keep digging," ordered the detectives, who now suspected they were standing on a burial ground. "There's got to be more."

Down in the basement, crime scene technicians wearing rubber gloves were collecting and bagging various items as evidence. To search for traces of blood, they sprayed a chemical called Luminol, which glows a fluorescent blue when it comes in contact with blood. Amazingly, a large round area on the basement floor lit up, as did the inside of several buckets detectives found in Berdella's outside gardening shed.

This encouraged the investigators to search further. The evidence was mounting. It was only a matter of time, they thought, until they would start finding the remains of the men in the photographs.

Meanwhile, news made its way to Berdella at his shop that a naked man had jumped from his second-floor window and that police were searching his house. Amazingly, Berdella didn't run. Instead, he drove his Toyota Tercel straight to his home. Wearing a black button-down shirt, he walked right up to police, identified himself, and asked what was going on.

About the same time, detectives arrived at Berdella's shop. They couldn't believe their eyes as they approached his booth. Sitting on the front counter, clearly in view of everyone, were four human skulls.

Back at 4315 Charlotte Avenue, investigators told Berdella they had some questions. Had he captured, tortured, and raped Chris Bryson? Did he do the same thing to Jerry Howell and James Ferris? Whose skull did they uncover in his backyard? Who were the young men in the photographs? Was he a Satanist? How many people had he tortured and murdered? What did he do with the bodies?

Berdella listened patiently to their on-the-spot interrogation. He simply shook his head and said he didn't know what they were talking about, and he said he wanted a lawyer. End of questioning. In 1966, the U.S. Supreme Court ruled in a case called *Miranda* v.

Arizona that police must read criminal defendants their rights before questioning them, including the right to have a lawyer present during police questioning. If the police continue to interrogate a suspect after he or she has requested a lawyer, then any evidence that comes from that is inadmissible in court.

The detectives sent the human skulls and the vertebrae for testing to a forensic anthropologist at Kansas State University. They hoped to find out the age, race, and gender of the person to whom this skull once belonged, and how long the person might have been dead, as well as any information about how he or she died. But most of all, they hoped to use the dental records to learn this person's identity.

If Berdella wasn't talking, the same could not be said for all of his neighbors. Rumors were abundant and becoming stranger by the day. That Berdella was a serial killer and rapist was tame speculation compared to the word circulating on the streets of Kansas City. Some people were betting that Berdella had fed the human flesh to his two pet Chow dogs—a rumor fueled by reports that his pets refused to eat dog food. Then there was the discovery of unmarked meat in Berdella's freezer. Neighbors thought back to the meat dishes that Berdella brought to community cookouts and to share with other businesspeople he worked with. Could Berdella be a cannibal on top of everything else?

The rumors were given legitimacy by the remaining question: If Berdella had killed the several young men portrayed in the pictures, what did he do with their bodies? A search of the rest of the backyard and the entire front yard produced no more human remains. Neighbors and fellow merchants were finally put at ease when police announced that the meat found in Berdella's freezer was, in fact, beef.

Stumped, the Kansas City police department created a special, twelve-person Robert Berdella task force. They redoubled their efforts, reinterviewing all of Berdella's neighbors and those who worked around him. But they focused heavily on the young men who worked the barren streets of downtown Kansas City. Known as "chicken hawks," the men were usually between eighteen and twenty-five years of age. Most were homeless, without jobs, living day-to-day. A number of them were bisexual and addicted to drugs. They would walk the streets hoping to be spotted by another man or woman or couple who offered money or drugs in return for sexual services.

The detectives who questioned the chicken hawks came to one quick conclusion: Robert Berdella frequently drove through the area seeking dates. And the police were amazed at how many of the young men were long aware of the rumors that he was dangerous. But still there was no concrete evidence to prove in a court of law that Berdella had actually killed anyone. Detectives were getting frustrated.

Within a couple of days, the forensic scientists at Kansas State University finished their experiments on the two skulls found at Berdella's home. Using chemical dating tests, researchers estimated that the skull found in the backyard was that of a male who was between twenty-five and thirty-six years old when he died. They believed he had been dead for as little as six weeks or as much as ten months. The scientists also said the vertebrae discovered in the backyard with the first skull displayed evidence of knife and saw marks.

The skull found in Berdella's home appeared to be that of a twenty-one- to thirty-two-year-old male. The researchers matched the teeth found in the envelope with the second skull. They estimated the death of this second male had occurred at least eighteen months earlier. However, a cause of death could not be determined in either case.

That same day, the police crime laboratory reported that there was human blood, human flesh, body tissue, and pubic hairs recovered from a chain saw seized in Berdella's basement.

Meanwhile, detectives were showing some of the Polaroid photographs found in Berdella's house to a few of the street hustlers in

Kansas City where Berdella used to regularly patrol. Some of the young men were hesitant to cooperate at first, but eventually a few names kept surfacing: Todd Stoops, Robert Sheldon, Larry Pearson, and Mark Wallace.

All of these men were missing. No one had seen them in months, maybe years. Investigators ran each of the names through their own police files and through the national computer system operated by the FBI. They were able to locate relatives of each of the men that they identified. More important, they were able to find the names of the doctors and dentists who had previously treated each of the men. Dental records were on the way.

Within a couple of days, researchers assisting the police announced a huge break: the dental records of Larry Pearson matched the remains found at Berdella's house. Combined with the photographs showing Pearson being tortured and raped in Berdella's house, prosecutors felt they had enough evidence to officially bring a murder charge.

The next day, Berdella was brought into the Kansas City Circuit Court to be arraigned on the charge of first-degree murder. The arraignment, or probable cause hearing, as it is known in some states, is a mere formality. It's a court hearing in which the prosecutors are required to read the charges and announce whether they would support the defendant being released on bail pending trial. In this case, the prosecutor obviously objected to any bail, insisting that Berdella remain in police custody until trial because of the seriousness of the charges.

The arraignment, as noted earlier, is also the time when the person charged with the crime enters an initial plea. Again, this is mostly a formality. Normally, the defense attorney representing the person charged will announce that the client is pleading not guilty and then seek a specific bail amount. But even at this traditionally boring court hearing, this case took a weird spin.

256

"At this time, it's the defendant's intention to enter a plea of guilty, as charged, to murder in the first degree," said Public Defender Patrick Berrigan.

The courtroom was stunned.

For the past thirty-five years, I have served as a prosecutor, coroner, medical examiner, and expert witness in thousand and thousands of criminal cases, but never have I witnessed a murder suspect plead guilty at the arraignment. It's simply unheard of. Berdella's decision to plead guilty caught the prosecutors off guard. Prosecutors had planned on filing notice with the court clerk later that week that they would seek the death penalty against the defendant. But this plea was a preemptive move. By agreeing to plead guilty to the crime of murder in the first degree, Berdella was automatically accepting the sentence of life in prison without the possibility of parole.

The law requires prosecutors to notify the court of their intention to seek the death penalty *prior* to a trial or even a plea. However, the same law says prosecutors should be given adequate time to determine if the first-degree murder case warrants capital punishment. The question was, how would prosecutors respond? Would they fight the guilty plea in order to seek capital punishment?

After a quick meeting with the senior lawyers in the Kansas City prosecutor's office, they announced they would not oppose Berdella's guilty plea and sentence to life without parole. Their reasoning was simple and very sound: they knew they would have more chances to seek the death penalty against Berdella. By accepting Berdella's guilty plea, they were guaranteed he would spend the remainder of his life on earth behind bars. And by pleading guilty, Berdella was waiving any right he had to appeal.

Missouri circuit judge Alvin Randall was also in shock. He told Berdella to sit in the witness chair. "Raise your right hand and be sworn," the judge said. "Do you swear to tell the truth, the whole truth, and nothing but the truth, so help you God?"

257

"I do," Berdella responded. He showed no sign of emotion whatsoever.

For the next fifteen minutes, Berrigan asked his client a series of questions.

Berrigan: Would you state your full name?

Berdella: Robert Andrew Berdella Jr.

Berrigan: What is your date of birth?

Berdella: January 31, 1949.

Berrigan: I'm going to ask you some questions pertaining to what it is that occurred on August 5, 1987, in Jackson County, Missouri. First, on that particular date, where were you living?

Berdella: At 4315 Charlotte Avenue.

Berrigan: Did you at that time know a person by the name of Larry W. Pearson?

Berdella: Yes.

Berrigan: Was he present in your house on that date?

Berdella: Yes.

Berrigan: Did you knowingly cause Mr. Pearson's death by asphyxiating him?

Berdella: Yes.

Berrigan: Could you tell the courtroom briefly what occurred?

Berdella: I put a plastic bag over his head, secured it with a rope and allowed him to suffocate.

Berrigan: Did you realize what you were doing?

Berdella: Yes.

Berrigan: Did you know that it would result in the death of Mr. Pearson?

Berdella: Yes.

Berrigan: Did you know at that time that what you did was against the law?

Berdella: Yes.

Within a few days, the crime laboratory had identified the second skull found in Berdella's house as that of Robert Sheldon. Prosecutors informed Berdella's lawyers that new murder charges were being prepared. This time, though, the prosecutors officially notified the court that they were planning to seek the death penalty. When Berdella was brought into court to face arraignment on this second murder charge, there was no surprise plea. He pleaded "not guilty" and a trial date was set.

A few days later, lawyers for Berdella approached prosecutors. They were interested in striking a deal. The defense attorneys knew that the police were having a difficult time developing evidence against Berdella on any of the additional cases. As a result, the families of several missing young men were frustrated and outraged. They wanted to know what happened to their sons.

The deal Berdella offered was simple: he would confess to everything he had done, give law enforcement details for every crime, and agree to plead guilty to each. In return, he wanted two things. First, he asked prosecutors to drop their request for the death penalty and agree to recommend that Berdella be sentenced to life in prison without parole. Second, he wanted prosecutors to end their bid to seize Berdella's house under state forfeiture laws.

Obviously, prosecutors were suspicious. They worried that they were being tricked. What if Berdella had kidnapped and killed dozens of young men? What if he had done the same to children? If either were true, the public would be outraged at prosecutors for agreeing to such a plea arrangement. At the same time, there was no guarantee that police would ever be able to put together enough evidence to charge Berdella with the murder of additional men. The deal being offered by Berdella would at least allow the victims' families to know for sure what happened and would allow the families to bury their loved ones, and it would give everyone a finality in a case that could cause doubt and pain for years.

To protect themselves, prosecutors wanted to know how many victims were involved. Now defense attorneys were on the spot. They didn't want to reveal any information their client had given them without a guarantee for a deal. In their next meeting, the defense attorneys told prosecutors the number of victims was no more than six.

After serious thought and heated debate, prosecutors made the decision to accept the deal. Both sides agreed that Berdella's full disclosure should not happen in open court. Instead, it would take place in a conference room in the basement of the local jail. And so it did. The room was small. The walls were tan cinder block. On one wall hung a blackboard, and three windows covered with brown paper lined another wall. Folding tables and chairs were brought in to accommodate all those assembled for the hearing.

Shortly after 9 A.M. on the morning of December 13, two prosecutors, Pat Hall and Albert Riederer, and two police detectives, Troy Cole and Albert DeValkenaere, walked into the room. Berdella and his two lawyers, Berrigan and Rogers, were already there. An official court stenographer was also present to record every word. For the next three days, Berdella answered every question posed to him.

Yes, he had kidnapped, drugged, tortured, raped, and murdered six young men. He told them how he had met each one and what he had done to them. Berdella also dismissed many of the rumors about him. No, he was not involved in devil worshiping, nor had he fed human flesh or bones to his dogs or put them in any food.

Berdella's sworn deposition took three days. Both sides issued press releases. The district attorney announced that Berdella had confessed to everything as part of a plea agreement. The two sides agreed that the following Monday, December 19, Berdella would make an official appearance in court to plead guilty to the five additional murders. On four of the five counts, the agreement was that Berdella would plead to second-degree murder. In the case of Robert Sheldon, Berdella agreed to plead guilty to first-degree murder. Prosecutors never explained why they chose to do it this way.

Once Berdella was safely secured in prison for the remainder of his life, his legal troubles would continue. The mother of Todd Stoops filed a wrongful-death lawsuit against Berdella. Of course, Berdella's financial fortune, such as it was, was not the real target: it was the insurance company that held his homeowner's policy.

It was at this point that I became involved in the case. The lawyers for the Stoops family needed a forensic pathologist to review all of the records in the case and determine how each victim died. But most important, the lawyers wanted to know if Berdella actually intended to kill Todd Stoops or if Stoops died unintentionally.

For two weeks in August 1992, I mulled over the records that the lawyers sent to me. As I stated earlier, the information was rather scant. Because no bodies were ever retrieved, there were no autopsy reports. All I had to go on were the photographs Berdella had taken of his victims, the lengthy diary Berdella kept, and Berdella's three-day sworn statement. While the basic circumstances about how Berdella had captured and killed his victims were known, the in-depth details were completely secret. The sworn deposition given by Berdella, which had been provided to me earlier, had not been made public.

On September 2, 1992, I sent my official report to Steven Harrell, a Springfield, Missouri, lawyer working on the case for the Stoops family. My goal in this report was to assemble the key pieces of evidence together in a manner that would tell the story of what happened. Here are excerpts from my report:

Clinical Summary

Mr. Todd Stoops was twenty-three years old at the time of his death on July 1, 1986. He was one of six young men who were held captive and killed in the residence of Mr. Robert Berdella, a forty-year-old homosexual.

Mr. Berdella had purchased a homeowner's insurance policy from Economy Fire and Casualty Company that provided him with liability insurance coverage. The law in Missouri would seemingly allow liability insurance coverage for Berdella if he did not expect or intend Stoops to die when he performed the acts which ultimately caused Stoops's death.

Berdella denied any satanic activity. He admitted using drugs to attract young men who were "bisexual or gay." He said he obtained the drugs from a veterinary supply house under the pretext of using them as tranquilizers for his dogs. Berdella suggested that he used the injections to basically immobilize his victims as sex objects.

Mr. Berdella gave a three-volume sworn statement from December 13 to 15, 1988, as part of a plea bargain for life imprisonment instead of the death penalty. He gave a detailed account of the circumstances of the deaths of his six victims. All the deaths occurred in his house at 4315 Charlotte Avenue, Kansas City, Missouri. Berdella dismembered the bodies, wrapped them in newspapers, put the parts into trash bags, and set them out on the curb to be picked up on Monday morning garbage collection dates.

The first victim, Jerry Holwell, died on July 5, 1984. Holwell was the son of the owner of a shop near the flea market store operated by Berdella. Berdella started to have a sexual relationship with Holwell in April 1984. He had helped Holwell pay for a lawyer, but Holwell refused to pay him back. At approximately 5:30 P.M. the night before, Berdella picked Holwell up at the young man's father's shop and took him home. Holwell passed out after Berdella gave him Valium, Triavil, and two Quaaludes.

262

Berdella repeatedly sodomized Holwell; he raped him with a carrot or a cucumber; injected Holwell with acepromazine and chlorpromaine. Berdella left Holwell bound when he went to work. Upon his return, he repeated the injections. When Holwell fought the restraints, Berdella slapped him with a metal ruler. Holwell vomited.

Jerry Holwell died at approximately 10 P.M. on July 5, 1984. Berdella felt that Holwell had gagged on the medications or asphyxiated from his vomit. Berdella hung him up by his feet "to drain the blood." He indicated that he did not intentionally torture the victim—it was to just control his captive. Berdella took photographs before he dismembered the body with cooking and boning knives and a chain saw. He had four or five bags for the body parts and separate bags for the clothes, drugs, and instruments he had used. Berdella watched as the trash was picked up from the curb. He made notes one or two weeks later.

Robert Sheldon had been known to Berdella since he had stayed in Berdella's house on three different occasions prior to this episode. Following an argument with the girl he was staying with, Sheldon appeared on Berdella's front porch with his tote bag on April 10, 1985. Berdella indicated that he was not sexually attracted to Sheldon. He kept him captive until April 14. In addition to sodomy, Berdella injected Drano into Sheldon's left eye. He also put a tattoo on Sheldon's left shoulder and filled his ears with caulking material.

Berdella performed acupuncture on Sheldon's fingertips. He administered strong whacks to the victim's head and back of the neck with a rubber mallet. He used piano wires to damage Sheldon's hands. In the photographs he took of Sheldon, Berdella included himself as a documentation and trophy.

On April 14, 1985, when Berdella came home from work, he found Paul Cooper on the roof of his house doing some tree work. Since he knew Cooper would come into the house to use the bathroom, Berdella put a trash bag over Sheldon's head and tied it with a sash or rope, causing him to suffocate. He took a photograph first. Later that evening, Berdella dismembered the body in the tub, wrapped the pieces, and stored them in the basement. For some unknown reason, he stuck the head in the freezer for a couple of days, and then buried it in the backyard.

Mark Wallace was about twenty or twenty-one years old. He helped mow Berdella's lawn. On June 22, 1985, during a rainstorm, Berdella found Wallace intoxicated in his tool shed. Berdella invited Wallace into the house, then gagged him, injected him with drugs, and sodomized him. He clubbed Wallace with a rubber mallet. Berdella applied electric shock to Wallace's shoulder three times and punctured the young man's back with needles.

At 5 P.M., when Berdella returned from work, Wallace was sitting up, trying to untie the ropes and wires. He started screaming for help, so Berdella injected him in the neck and buttocks and put a rag over his mouth. He then dismembered Wallace with a safety razor, boning knife, and bone saw. Berdella discarded the bags of body parts for a Monday morning pickup by the garbage truck.

On September 26, 1985, Walter Ferris asked to stay at Berdella's house. Berdella gave Ferris two Valiums, Advil, Triavil, and Seconal. They ate in the bedroom. At 9 P.M., Ferris passed out. Berdella went through his torture of injections, electric shock, and sodomy. He noticed that one of Ferris's arm veins was inflamed, and that he was feverish, vomiting, and shaking. Nevertheless, Berdella continued the injections and sodomy. He gave Ferris a total of 60 cc. of ketamine and 70.5 cc. of chlorpromazine. Ferris died around midnight on September 27, 1985.

Berdella bled the body in the bathtub by incising the blood vessels in the groin and the antecubital regions. He disposed of the body parts as usual.

The sixth victim, Larry Pearson, was killed after Todd Stoops. Berdella met Pearson, a male prostitute, in April or May of 1987. Berdella took Pearson captive on June 23, 1987.

Because Pearson was "very cooperative," he lasted for one and a half months. Berdella broke Pearson's hands to incapacitate him. He kept him as his sex slave. In the last week, Berdella placed a dog collar and leash on Pearson's neck. One day, when Pearson tried fighting back, Berdella hit his slave on the back of the head and "knocked him out." After his death and dismemberment, Berdella put Pearson's head in a plastic bag and stored it in the freezer. One week later, Berdella removed Sheldon's head from where he had buried it, and then buried Pearson's head. He later removed the teeth from Sheldon's skull and cleaned them, keeping the skull in his closet.

Todd Stoops was the youngest of four brothers. He also had a sister four years younger than he. He was athletic and competitive while growing up. Mr. Joe Edward Stoops, Todd's father, was a sheet metal worker. He had separated from Todd's mother in the summer of 1981, and they were divorced in December 1982, when Todd was nineteen years old. Mr. Stoops did not see much of Todd from 1982 until his death in 1986. Most of 1983 and 1984, Mr. Stoops had to work out of town for months at a time in Colorado, Nevada, and New Hampshire. Todd spent Thanksgiving 1982 with his father and his new wife. Mrs. Betty Haste, Todd's mother, drove a truck with her new husband.

In 1984, Mr. Stoops posted bond for Todd who was charged with marijuana possession. He visited Todd at the municipal farm several times when he was incarcerated. In March or April 1986, Todd called his father and told him that he had been in Oklahoma, had found God, and was getting things straightened up in his life.

Todd had numerous previous arrests. A total of eleven are listed, starting on December 30, 1981, for possession of marijuana, larceny, concealed weapon, obstructing an officer, disorderly conduct, prostitution, and assault. The last arrest for possession of marijuana was on July 5, 1986. He also had a record of two episodes of escape from the municipal farm.

Berdella testified that he had known Todd since the spring of

1984. Todd and Lisa, Todd's wife, had moved on two separate occasions into Berdella's house. The first time was reported to be in exchange for sexual favors from Todd, with Lisa's knowledge. Berdella was always sexually attracted to Todd. To show his feelings, Berdella bailed Todd out of jail.

On June 17, 1986, Berdella went to a place where male prostitutes hang out. He found Todd, who desperately wanted a shot of Ritalin and Talwin. Todd needed $13 and offered to "do anything you want."

Berdella got the Ritalin and Talwin for Todd, and then took him to his house. After feeding Todd, Berdella drugged him. The daily notes kept by Berdella on Todd Stoops indicated that on the first day that Todd was held captive, he was given two tetracycline capsules ("doctored" capsules, in fact, containing sedatives) between 1 P.M. and 2 P.M., and again at 4 P.M. on Tuesday, June 16, 1986.

Early in Todd's captivity, Berdella inserted his fist into the victim's rectum, known as "fisting." There was no heavy bleeding at first. Later, Berdella noted a large, dark, thick bloody mass (which Berdella's notes indicate began at about 6 A.M.). There were more episodes of slight bleeding, but "the rupture did not heal." Todd then developed a fever and shakes. Berdella administered ampicillin, tetracycline, and penicillin, which he had available for his dogs. He administered these antibiotics in the form of ointments and injections.

Berdella continued the sexual assaults, the use of electric shock, whipping, injection of Drano in the eyes "to permanently blind him for long-term captivity," injection of Drano into the voice box to prevent Todd from being able to scream.

Todd appeared dehydrated in his last days. Berdella moved him to the third floor on June 30. He kept a log, consisting of four pages, and took numerous photographs. Anal bleeding and discharge were noted on June 27: "rupture of the wall." Berdella bent Todd's fingers, and gagged his mouth with a piano wire that cut badly into his flesh. Todd eventually died on July 1, 1986. Berdella dismembered the body on a board across the bathtub with the use of a safety razor, boning knife, and bone saw. He stored the body parts in the basement for six days until Monday when they were picked up as trash.

Shelly L. Tepper, M.D., a board-certified forensic pathologist, and associate medical examiner for Jackson County, testified that Todd Stoops died as a complication of an anal wall tear.

As a result, Todd's rectum became infected. Bacteria and feces in the peritoneal cavity were manifested clinically as a fever. There was tightening of the abdominal muscles. The cause of Todd Stoops's death was septic shock. Eighty reproductions of the Polaroid photographs taken of Todd Stoops during his captivity by Berdella had been submitted for examination.

Medicolegal Questions

What was the nature and extent of Todd Stoops's rectal injury?

Berdella's confession detailed the sexual assault. He also described some anal bleeding, which was followed by a large, dark, bloody mass. More anal bleeding was documented in Berdella's notes. There was persistent anal discharge that required some routine change in dressings. Berdella also indicated that the rupture did not heal itself, despite his application of an antibiotic ointment.

What complications followed the rectal injury?

The rupture of the anal opening and the rectum caused an infection at the site of the injury. There was contamination of the traumatized area by urine and fecal material. Berdella described the presence of a "diaper rash." Fever and chills presented as the hallmark of a systemic infection. Berdella even noticed that Todd became dehydrated. There was prominent thirst, and Berdella tried to administer antibiotics and fluid. Death was a result of sepsis.

Was the death intentional?

Berdella admitted to sexual abuse and torture. The acts were intentional. He immobilized his victims through the administration of drugs by injection to have full control over them. Berdella indicated that he wanted to keep the victims alive as his sexual slaves. With the last two victims, Todd Stoops and Larry Pearson, Berdella had held them captive for much longer periods than his other victims, because these two "cooperated" with Berdella's treatments. Berdella confessed to injecting drain cleaner into their eyes "to permanently blind them for long-term captivity."

Berdella administered antibiotics when he suspected that his victim had some fever. He gave Todd ampicillin, tetracycline, and penicillin. Dr. Tepper suggested that the antibiotics Berdella gave were ineffective because the most likely infecting organism was an anaerobic bacteria. While ampicillin may be ineffective against anaerobic bacteria, both penicillin and tetracycline could be appropriate in proper dosages against these anaerobic organisms.

However, it was very likely that Todd had a mixed infection. Complicating urinary tract organisms would have been aerobic. Multiple resistant organisms were most likely involved. From the notes, Berdella treated Todd Stoops five times with various forms of antibiotics.

In my opinion, Berdella did not intentionally kill Todd Stoops.

Opinion

Following my evaluation and analysis of all the materials, it is my professional opinion, based upon a reasonable degree of medical certainty, that the sexual abuse and torture of Todd Stoops by Robert Berdella were intentional acts committed by Berdella when he held his victim captive and incapacitated him with injected drugs.

The rupture of the anorectal canal through a homosexual act of fisting was unexpected and unplanned. The rupture was com-

plicated by an overwhelming infection that ascended anatomi-
cally to produce peritonitis and sepsis, which eventually caused
this young man's death.

There were definite, genuine attempts to treat the infection.
However, the treatment was inadequate and inappropriate, and
therefore, Todd Stoops's death was not prevented.

I sent my ten-page report to the lawyers involved in the case.
My findings were particularly important to the lawyers for Ms.
Haste in pursuing their case against the insurance company. Bear in
mind that Berdella's insurance policy would not cover Todd
Stoops's death if he died as the result of an intentional homicide.
But that was not my finding. In my scientific opinion, Stoops died
because of Berdella's negligence.

True, Berdella intentionally kidnapped and tortured his victims.
And he knew they would eventually die from his actions. That evidence is certainly enough to convict him in a criminal case for first-
degree murder. However, that is not true in a civil case like this.
What the Stoopses' family lawyer had to show was that Berdella
did not want Stoops to die, that he tried to keep Stoops alive, and
that Berdella's actions failed as the result of negligence.

In my scientific expert opinion, the evidence in this case shows
that Todd Stoops died when he did because Berdella administered
the wrong antibiotic. Berdella thought that by treating Stoops with
the antibiotics, he would be keeping his victim alive. But he was
wrong, and as a result of Berdella's mistake, Todd Stoops died. By
definition, that is negligence.

Indeed, this was a very novel argument by the lawyers for Betty
Ann Haste, Stoops's mother. It also happened to be scientifically
and medically correct and true.

Once I made my report, I expected one of two things to happen.
First, the case would either move forward toward trial and the

lawyers on both sides would want to meet with me to take my sworn deposition, or the two sides would settle the lawsuit out of court before trial.

The latter is what happened in the case of *Betty Ann Haste* v. *Economy Fire and Casualty Insurance Company*. The pressure on the insurance company to settle became more intense in 1993 when the Missouri Court of Appeals ruled in 1992 that Berdella's policy was valid and that the insurance company could be held liable, not only for the original verdict, but also for interest accruing on the judgment. According to court officials, the interest on the $5 billion judgment was amounting to $600,000 a day.

In 1994, lawyers in the case told me that Economy Fire and Casualty had agreed to settle the lawsuit for $2.5 million. The lawyers told me that it was much more than they thought they would get. The lawsuit was a long shot to begin with, and the $5 billion verdict had gained national attention.

I must say that in four decades of investigating strange and unexplained homicides, and performing thousands and thousands of autopsies, I have never participated in a case so outrageous, and with such bizarre legal questions, as the case of Robert Berdella.

Like Jeffrey Dahmer, Berdella died in prison. On October 9, 1992, prison officials found Berdella in his cell, dead from a heart attack. A quote from a fellow inmate, in the *Kansas City Star* of October 10, 1992, summed up the entire Berdella case: "There was no grief at his death—there wasn't a frown in the house."

Chapter Nine

HEAVY METAL MURDER

The Curious Demise of Robert Curley

WHEN ROBERT CURLEY FIRST ENTERED Wilkes-Barre General Hospital in August 1991, he complained of intermittent leg pains, numbness, weakness, nausea, and burning in the soles of his feet and palms of his hands. The symptoms had been coming on for more than a week before Curley, a thirty-two-year-old electrician in the blue-collar town in eastern Pennsylvania, was admitted to the hospital.

Doctors initially were puzzled. Curley had a family history of heart disease—his father had died at fifty-two of a heart attack and a brother had died at thirty-two of another heart ailment. But many of the signs Curley exhibited weren't connected to heart troubles. He repeatedly vomited, and the pain in his body was so severe that Curley was screaming in agony. Hospital staff observed Curley for three and a half days, and his condition seemed to stabilize, even

271

improve slightly. When he was discharged August 29, it was with the tentative diagnosis of Guillain-Barre syndrome. Named after two Frenchmen, the disease affects certain nerves in the body. Although it can be associated with people who've had some sort of vaccination, it is often unclear what brings on this sometimes fatal affliction.

Once Curley was back home, however, his health didn't improve. The searing pain in Curley's feet returned to the point that he could no longer walk. Soon he grew weaker and became bedridden. Nine days after being released from the hospital, an ambulance took him back. This time, testing revealed mild dehydration and a low potassium level, which suggested something possibly involving the kidneys. Doctors noticed other symptoms that indicated their initial diagnosis of Guillain-Barre syndrome might not be accurate. One had to do with Curley's hair—it was falling out. The observation of alopecia (hair loss) was made September 10, three days after Curley was readmitted. The day after that a biopsy of his stomach showed inflammation, or gastritis.

Now his physicians began to consider the possibility that Curley was suffering from some sort of heavy metal exposure. On September 16, he was transferred to the larger Hershey Medical Center, where staff thought that he appeared as if he were a chemotherapy patient. Curley underwent testing for the heavy metals— arsenic, lead, mercury, and cadmium—but all the results were negative. A neurological exam also turned up nothing, as did other diagnostic tests.

Despite the negative findings, Curley continued to have severe problems. His hair loss worsened. He became increasingly confused and agitated, and often combative with hospital staff. He yelled and threw his food. Eventually, leather restraints had to be imposed to control Curley's outbursts. A psychiatrist who saw Curley on September 19 prescribed Haldol and Ativan, two drugs used to treat people with mental agitation or emotional distress.

Without a firm handle on what was causing Curley's difficulties, the hospital was reduced to treating his symptoms.

There were some indications that this approach was working. On September 21, Curley's agitation began to decrease and he was more lucid. He had improved so much by the next day that his brother brought pizza and orange drink to the hospital, and his wife and sister also visited. But Curley's recovery was short-lived. That night he became very agitated, his temperature spiked, and his heart rhythm was tachycardic, or beating faster than normal. At eight o'clock the next morning, Robert Curley went into cardiac arrest. Doctors repeatedly shocked his system with a defibrillator—eight times in all—and eventually were able to resuscitate him. They placed Curley on a ventilator, but he remained unresponsive and in a coma.

Curley's condition continued to worsen, but on September 25, his physicians finally got a break. Test results of Curley's urine showed he had more than nine hundred times the expected amount of the heavy metal thallium in his system. Suddenly, his symptoms—the hair loss, the nerve deficiencies, the gastritis—all made sense. Doctors immediately started Curley on a heavy metal chelator, a chemical designed to absorb the heavy metals in his body and flush them out. But by then, it was too late. Curley's condition did not improve, and he remained in a coma. His wife, Joann, agreed to remove life support September 27.

Within days, the government's Occupational Safety and Health Administration (OSHA) sent an investigator to Curley's most recent work site, a building being renovated at Wilkes University. Curley had been on the job since mid-May, and officials discovered five bottles of thallium salts in the stockroom of the chemistry laboratory where he had been working. The OSHA investigator took air samples and wiped the room's surfaces, but found no traces of thallium. Additionally, thirteen of Curley's coworkers who spent time in the same areas were tested and showed no signs of thallium exposure.

273

Nearly a month after Curley's death, police began their own investigation and eventually questioned the other employees. One theory authorities considered was that someone wanted to play a prank on Curley by putting something in his iced tea. Detectives wondered whether pranksters may have mistaken the thallium found at the site for similar-sounding Valium, the tranquilizer. Then in December, the coroner ruled Curley's death a homicide, based partly on the conclusion that the levels of thallium in his blood and urine were so high he had to have ingested the poison rather than inhaled it or absorbed it through his skin.

Because he sought treatment, suicide was ruled out. Detectives from the Pennsylvania State Police joined the case, and a task force was created to investigate. But the case still stalled. His wife hired an attorney to file a notice that she planned to file a civil lawsuit against Wilkes University in connection with his death. But in the criminal case, years went by and produced no new leads, no signs to help detectives figure out who killed Robert Curley.

●　•　ͺ

In March 1996, I got a phone call from Peter Paul Olszewski Jr., the district attorney of Luzerne County, Pennsylvania. I was familiar with Olszewski, having testified in two murder cases in his county, in 1990 and 1994. I happened to be working with the defense in both cases, but like all dedicated professionals, Olszewski didn't hold that against me. Actually, my history in Wilkes-Barre goes back further, to 1969, when I testified in the city on behalf of prosecutors in the Mary Jo Kopechne case. As many will recall, Kopechne, a twenty-eight-year-old political campaign worker, was riding in a car driven by Sen. Edward Kennedy in July 1969 in Massachusetts. She drowned after the vehicle ran off a bridge on Chappaquiddick Island. Massachusetts prosecutors wanted permission to exhume her body, which had been buried where she grew up in Luzerne County, to find out more about how she died. I had planned to do the autopsy, but after a hearing on the issue, a judge in Wilkes-Barre denied the request.

Now on the phone with Olszewski, he told me about a curious case involving a man who had died of thallium poisoning. No one had been arrested at that point, but officials were closing in on a suspect. He asked me if I would review the pathological and toxicological findings, along with other evidence, that led investigators to believe they had identified the person responsible for the crime.

My first step was to find more information about thallium. While I certainly knew that the heavy metal was carcinogenic, thallium poisoning was not something I routinely came across in my job as coroner or consultant on other cases. The same went for arsenic, cadmium, lead, mercury, and many other metals. Even though it is not common to find thallium and similar heavy metals, good toxicology laboratories, such as the one in Allegheny County, test for them in certain situations. Usually those screenings are conducted when there are suspicions of a drug death, but normal toxicology tests fail to turn up any toxic substances.

Thallium, I learned, was discovered in 1861 by the English chemist Sir William Crookes, who noticed a bright green line in the spectrum while examining samples of dust from a sulfuric acid industrial plant in a spectrograph. Crookes named the chemical element after the Greek word *thallos*, which means young green shoot or twig. For a time, thallium actually was used for medical purposes, much like arsenic. Doctors prescribed it as a treatment for scalp ringworm, syphilis, gonorrhea, and gout, but it eventually fell out of favor because of its toxicity.

Thallium later was used in rat poison, but U.S. production of it ended in 1972, and it was banned in this country in 1984, again because of its toxicity. The heavy metal is still used mainly in manufacturing electronic devices and switches. Thallium also is utilized as a depilatory agent in the glass and dye industries. Additionally, small amounts of thallium isotopes are employed in medical tests, especially stress tests and other cardiac exams, but the levels used are not dangerous.

The salts of thallium are odorless, colorless, and tasteless—desirable qualities for someone who wants to use it as a poison. The heavy metal can enter the body not only through ingestion, eating or drinking something contaminated, but also by inhaling it, or having it come in contact with the skin. Acute ingestion, that is, large amounts over a short time period, causes vomiting, diarrhea, and hair loss, and affects the nervous system, lungs, heart, liver, and kidneys. Exposure to smaller doses over an extended period also causes those symptoms, but the onset is more gradual.

Thallium can be found in minute levels in almost all people, perhaps more so in residents who live in the vicinity of coal-burning power plants. Generally speaking, a lethal dose can range from 0.5 grams to 1 gram. That's not a lot, considering a gram is about a quarter of a teaspoon.

I have heard of other heavy metal poisoning cases, although by no means are they a common occurrence. A famous, if entirely fictional, thallium poisoning was documented in Agatha Christie's 1952 mystery novel *The Pale Horse*. And recent testing on a lock of hair taken from French emperor Napoleon Bonaparte after his death in 1821 showed arsenic levels many times above normal. The tests were seen as proof of rumors that the British had slowly poisoned Napoleon while he was in exile on the tiny island of St. Helena off the African coast. However, further testing of Napoleon's hair taken at several different times in his life showed elevated arsenic levels many years prior to his exile. The most plausible explanation, according to scientists who conducted the follow-up tests, was that a hair product in the early nineteenth century typically contained arsenic.[1]

But poisoning by heavy metals such as thallium and arsenic—whether accidental or intentional—have been, by and large, isolated incidents, mostly because these types of toxins are not found in society nearly as much in the decades since insecticides and rodenticides containing them have been banned. That doesn't mean cases don't still happen, however.

A study of 292 homicidal poisonings between 1980 and 1989 noted those crimes are among the most difficult to detect and to bring charges against the killer. The study's authors, a member of the FBI Academy's behavioral science unit and two others, focused on four cases in which the poisoning was missed initially by both police and doctors. Interestingly, one involved a woman who fed her boyfriend arsenic-laced peanut butter milkshakes and banana pudding while he was in the hospital. Authorities later charged her with killing her first husband and poisoning another husband, who got sick on their honeymoon.

In another case, a Florida man was charged after tainting a neighboring family's Coca-Cola bottles with thallium because he didn't like them. The mother of the family died after spending several weeks in the hospital and was wrongly diagnosed with a nervous system disorder—not unlike the initial diagnosis in the Curley case.[2]

●　•　●

After looking through Curley's medical records for his hospital stays, I reviewed the autopsy, which Dr. M. L. Cowen performed the morning after Curley died. Dr. Cowen listed the cause of death as severe hypoxic encephalopathy, secondary to thallium poisoning. Hypoxic means the brain was getting decreased amounts of oxygen, while encephalopathy means pathological changes of the brain of a nonspecific nature. So even though there was no hemor-

277

rhage, tumor, or infection in the brain, it nonetheless was not normal. Curley's brain showed severe edema, or swelling, along with herniation, which occurs with pronounced brain swelling. Essentially, herniation means his brain, in search of a way to relieve the pressure, began to push down into an open area inside the skull where the spinal cord emerges from the cranial vault.

One of the first things police investigators did when they started their inquiry was search the house that Curley had shared with his wife of thirteen months and her four-year-old daughter from a previous marriage. Twenty-eight-year-old Joann Curley, née Steligo, did not object to officers scouring the home for clues, at which time they seized nearly one hundred items. Among the articles detectives took were thermoses, including one that Joann Curley said her husband used to bring iced tea with him to work. Tests on the thermoses were positive for thallium.

Authorities also conferred with medical consultants during the investigation. One of them was Dr. Ward Donovan, a clinical toxicologist at Hershey Medical Center, who had helped treat Robert Curley. He had done testing on Joann Curley and her daughter, both of whom showed elevated thallium levels. The results were unusual, but neither had what was considered toxic exposure, and further testing showed that the levels were decreasing, so doctors decided no treatment was necessary.

Dr. Donovan worked to determine when the Curleys first may have been exposed to thallium and came up with on or about August 16. Robert Curley died September 27. Dr. Donovan reached his conclusion based partly on information from Joann Curley, who said she had flulike symptoms August 16 and 17, and her husband experienced a similar illness the following two days. Robert Curley then showed signs of neurological problems on August 23.

But that evidence didn't help answer *how* Curley was exposed to thallium. Investigators initially had focused on the window of time immediately before Curley's hospital admittance, which seemed to fit with the theory that he somehow ingested the thallium from the Wilkes University job site. That avenue of investigation, however, seemed to be leading nowhere. Detectives and prosecutors turned to experts they had consulted in previous cases for ideas.

One of them was Dr. Fredric Rieders, a forensic toxicologist who ran his own laboratory, called National Medical Services, in Willow Grove, Pennsylvania. I've known Dr. Rieders for forty years, and he is considered one of the top forensic toxicologists in the nation. In fact, I've relied on his lab for toxicology work in many previous cases. During discussions with authorities, Dr. Rieders said he could do an analysis that could create a timeline, plotting the points of Curley's thallium exposure. But such testing required more samples than were taken from Curley during the original autopsy. His body would have to be exhumed.

Authorities approached Joann Curley with the idea, and she agreed. On August 23, 1994, my colleague Dr. Michael Baden, the notable forensic pathologist mentioned in earlier chapters, performed a second autopsy. This time, hair shafts from Curley's scalp, eyebrows, chest, and pubic area were taken. Baden also collected samples of toenails, fingernails, skin, and other tissues where heavy metals such as thallium are deposited.

Dr. Rieders assisted in the second autopsy. Once all the specimens were secured during the second postmortem examination, Dr. Rieders went to work. The main testing he conducted was segmental analyses of the hairs taken from Curley's scalp. The process allowed Dr. Rieders to create a chronology of thallium exposure in the last months of Curley's life. While the actual procedure is somewhat complex, the idea behind it is quite simple. Human head hair grows an average of one millimeter (0.04 inches) every 2.7 days. The samples taken from Curley's head were 122 millimeters long from root to tip, or roughly five inches. Therefore, the last 329 days of Curley's life, at least in terms of thallium levels, were recorded in the strands of his hair.

After washing the individual hairs, Dr. Rieders lined up four bundles and cut them from root to tip into twenty-five sections. The segments closest to the roots, which represented the time just before Curley died, were divided into one- and two-millimeter pieces. The next fourteen sections going out were cut at lengths of five millimeters each, and the final four pieces were divided into ten-millimeter segments. In essence, the farther away from the scalp, the longer the piece of hair. This was done because Dr. Rieders wanted to obtain as much specificity as possible relating to the days leading up to Curley's death. It would have been unnecessary, not to mention more costly and time consuming, to test the entire length of hair at one- or two-millimeter intervals.

Dr. Rieders was able to determine the levels of thallium in each tiny section by a process called atomic absorption spectrophotometry. After using a chemical method to break down each segment of bundled hair into individual atoms, he excited the atoms to the point that they absorbed energy. Everything from thallium to cocaine has a different rate of energy absorption, which can be measured. The procedure provides evidence not only of the presence of a substance like thallium but also of the quantity of the substance.

What the testing revealed was quite interesting. During the period between the end of October 1990 and the beginning of November, represented by the very tip of Curley's hair strands, the thallium level in his body was 0.5 parts per million (ppm). Twenty-seven days later, the thallium level was 3 ppm, six times the previous amount. The concentrations declined toward the end of 1990 and the beginning of the new year, but climbed even higher sometime in February. By March, Curley had 7 ppm of thallium in his system. Then, just as before, the levels slowly dropped during the following two and a half months. Another upswing was seen starting in the middle of May 1991, about the time Curley started his job at the university. By the end of August 1991, the thallium level in his body was at 8 ppm.

The number hit 9.5 ppm sometime during the first week of September 1991, and after it slipped to 3 ppm about a week later, the level began rising steadily until Curley's death. Interestingly, there was a massive spike that corresponded to the last two to four days of Curley's life. The final segment—basically the root of his hair—showed a thallium concentration of 26 ppm.

Hair from other parts of Curley's body, which had different average growth rates, showed similar patterns. Testing on his eyebrow hairs went back only about fifty-six days from his death. The thallium level at the tip end was 7 ppm, and the level at the root, the point closest to his death, was 20 ppm. Thallium also is deposited in a person's nails, and Curley's toenails revealed a level of 0.7 ppm at the oldest point in time. Since toenails have an average growth rate of 0.07 millimeters a day, and Curley's toenail sample was 18.2 millimeters long, that reading coincided with about 260 days prior to his death. In contrast, the root of Curley's toenail had a thallium level of 5.2 ppm.

The levels and time frames relating to Curley's scalp hair were then correlated with other aspects of his life. For example, in early to mid-May the thallium levels in Curley's system were 1.5 ppm, quite low compared to other times. As it turns out, Curley was on a fishing trip in Canada with friends between May 10 and 15.

Concentrations continued to rise upon his return and into the summer. There was a small dip of 1 ppm in mid-August—his first wedding anniversary was August 11—but when Curley was admitted for the first time to Wilkes-Barre General Hospital on August 26, the level was rising again. It reached 8 ppm at that time and 9.5 ppm about a week or so later, which generally coincided with Curley's second hospital admission on September 7.

From that date until his death, Curley was hospitalized, either at Wilkes-Barre or Hershey Medical Center. As would be expected, the next hair segment showed Curley's thallium level had dropped, and by sometime in early to mid-September it was at 3 ppm. However, in the last week or so of Curley's life, the toxic heavy metal readings in his body increased to 6 ppm, then 7.5 ppm, and finally to 26 ppm. The final reading was a bit misleading, though. I believed the huge jump was part of the body's excretion process, helped on in the final days by the chelating agent, which was flushing out the toxin. Curley's body was trying to get rid of the thallium every way it could, and that included through the hair roots.

Based on the test results, Dr. Rieders concluded the levels of thallium in Curley's body were enough to cause his death. "The results of the segmental analyses of hair and nails show several episodes of thallium introduction into Robert Curley, starting at least six months and possibly as long as eleven months before his death, with a last episode after his transfer to Hershey Medical Center in September of 1991," Rieders wrote in his report.[3]

I had to agree. The thallium level present in Curley's system during the last week of his life pointed strongly to an additional exposure while he was in the hospital. But when? Authorities focused on the evening of September 22, when Curley was well enough to have visitors, and to enjoy some pizza and soft drink. His wife, Joann, was alone with him at the end of the visit, and about an hour later, at 8:20 P.M., Curley's condition suddenly deteriorated. His temperature spiked, he became very agitated, and his heart was tachycardic (beating fast). Researching the issue, I learned that large doses of thallium initially can produce tachycardia.

Further evidence of a thallium ingestion at the hospital was found in Curley's gastrointestinal tract. Specimens of Curley's small and large intestines were taken during the second autopsy, which revealed thallium levels so high that they were astounding.

282

When describing the results of tests on Curley's lung and liver tissues, Dr. Rieders expressed the levels in parts per million. A sample from his lung had 3.9 ppm, while a liver sample had 1.2 ppm of thallium. However, the thallium concentrations found in the area of the small intestine closest to Curley's stomach right through to his colon were more than 1,000 times higher. That meant Dr. Rieders had to use *parts per thousand*, as opposed to parts per million. A section of the intestine nearest to the stomach had a thallium concentration of 4.1 ppk (parts per thousand), or 4,100 ppm.

I believed that the most likely time frame for Curley to have been exposed to the thallium was the evening of September 22, when he was conscious and relatively alert. He couldn't have ingested any from the morning of September 23 until his death, because he was in a coma. Curley's markedly reduced metabolism—including his gastrointestinal functions—would explain why thallium still was present in his small intestine at the time he died, about four days after ingestion. Normally, food passes through the stomach in about two hours, and liquids pass much quicker.

There were only a few people who could have supplied Curley with a dose of thallium during that period. At the top of the list was his wife, Joann Curley.

By the time I became involved in the case, detectives already had cast a suspicious eye on Curley's widow. I later learned from a probable cause affidavit in the case that they had good reasons.

One of the most basic questions investigators try to answer in a homicide case is who benefits from the victim's death. Often times that enrichment is monetary, and in the case of Robert Curley, police didn't have to look far for a fairly obvious explanation. Joann Curley was the sole beneficiary of her husband's life insurance and employment death benefits. Soon after the two were married in August 1990, Robert Curley changed beneficiaries from his mother to his new wife. After he died, Joann Curley collected nearly $297,000.

But that was not the only payout she received. Joann Curley's first husband was killed in a car accident in April 1988, eight months before she met Robert Curley. She filed a wrongful-death lawsuit, and the case went to trial on September 9, 1991, just days after her second husband was taken to the hospital for a second time. Friends and coworkers of Robert Curley said that before he became ill, he often spoke about spending portions of whatever funds Joann Curley was to recover to start his own electrical contracting business, go on vacation to Hawaii, and build a house. Robert Curley's brother, David, later told authorities Joann Curley was adamantly opposed to his plans.

There would have been plenty of money. On September 23, 1991, the day Robert Curley went into cardiac arrest and slipped into a coma from which he never recovered, Joann Curley settled her case against one of the defendants for $925,000. Two days later, the jury in the civil trial awarded her another $150,000 from the second defendant.

Detectives also focused on the thermoses Robert Curley took to work with him. Joann Curley told authorities early in the investigation that her husband always took a half-gallon Coleman thermos filled with iced tea to his job at Wilkes University. He brought home whatever was left over at the end of the day and continued to drink from it in the evening. Testing of that thermos showed signs of thallium.

Investigators eventually obtained a total of three thermoses from the Curley residence. In addition to the Coleman, they gathered a pint-size Stanley thermos and a quart-size Stanley thermos. When detectives interviewed Joann Curley in October 1991, less than a month after her husband's death, she said that Robert Curley never took either of the Stanley thermoses to work with him. Curiously, the pint-size thermos also tested positive for thallium.

Soon after the testing results came back, a local newspaper

reported that two of Robert Curley's thermoses showed signs of thallium contamination. About two weeks later, Joann Curley told police that she remembered pouring iced tea from her husband's Coleman thermos into the Stanley pint-size one and bringing it to Robert Curley at the hospital August 27, 1991. Curley's hospital roommate at the time later told detectives Joann Curley showed up with a thermos that was at least two quarts and with a handle—characteristics authorities said better described the Coleman thermos.

While much of the later investigation focused on finding evidence that might link Joann Curley to the crime, detectives also spent time eliminating other possible sources of Robert Curley's thallium exposure. The most obvious origin seemed to be the thallium found at the Wilkes University lab. Samples from the five jars of thallium salt located near the work area were tested to see if they were similar to the thallium Curley had been exposed to. They weren't. But perhaps even more compelling was Dr. Rieders's timeline, which clearly showed high levels of thallium in Curley's system as far back as late November 1990, and most definitely by early March 1991. That was at least two months before Curley started working at the college.

The timeline also was helpful in excluding other people as suspects. Whoever poisoned Robert Curley needed to have access not only to him, but also to his food and drink during the many periods in which the thallium levels in his body increased dramatically. Although investigators initially focused on some of Robert Curley's coworkers, none of them had the access required during the exposure periods.

Detectives used the same method to eliminate his friends and family members such as his mother, brother, sister, and sister-in-law. They may have been around him during some of the times, but not all of the times he grew sicker. That left one person: Joann Curley.

● • ●

Among the questions prosecutor Olszewski had asked me to consider was when Joann Curley was exposed to thallium. At one point after her husband's death, Joann Curley called Dr. Donovan, the Hershey clinical toxicologist, while he was in Toronto at a convention, and conveyed her anxieties about the concentrations of thallium in and around her home. She insisted that she be tested, and those tests were done October 3 and 7. Joann Curley had a blood thallium level of 13.6 nanograms per milliliter (ng/ml) and a urine thallium level of 172 micrograms per liter (µg/L). To put that in perspective, Robert Curley's urine thallium level was 1828 µg/L on September 19 and 4860 µg/L on September 27. It seemed likely to me that Joann Curley intentionally ingested a little bit of thallium after her husband died as a way to deflect suspicion away from her. That also could explain why low levels of thallium were found in her daughter as well.

Beginning in early September 1996 and then again at the end of November, stories in the local media reported the imminent arrest of Joann Curley. Though the timing was off, the reporters were on the right track. On December 12, Pennsylvania State Police arrested Joann Curley on charges of first-degree murder.

The arrest drew an enormous amount of attention from both the media and the community. At a bail hearing later in December in the Luzerne County courthouse, more than one hundred people packed into the courtroom of common pleas judge Correale Stevens. Television cameramen surrounded Joann Curley as she was led in handcuffs and shackles into the court.[4] The district attorney opposed any bail, and Judge Stevens denied the defense's request, ruling that prosecutors had submitted enough details in a fifteen-page summary of the evidence to warrant Joann Curley's continued detainment.

My participation in the case culminated in a two-day preliminary hearing held January 31 and February 3, 1997. The purpose of the hearing before Wilkes-Barre district justice Martin Kane was to determine whether prosecutors had enough evidence against Curley to bind the case over for trial. Olszewski wanted me to testify about the segmental analyses conducted by Dr. Rieders and my other conclusions.

On the witness stand, Olszewski had me go through Robert Curley's medical condition and problems during his hospital stays, as well as the initial autopsy findings. Then the district attorney brought out a chart, somewhat like a timeline, that laid out the thallium levels in Robert Curley's hair at different points in time. The chart had columns denoting a particular section of hair, identified by how many millimeters it was away from the root; the days prior to death; a specific date; and a "window of opportunity," which was one week ahead and one week behind the previous column's specific date. The window was used to allow for variations in individual growth rates of hair.

Olszewski asked me about the segments furthest in time from Curley's death in November 1990, when the thallium level went from 0.5 ppm to 3.5 ppm.

"During that period of time, there has been one or more ingestions of a significant amount of thallium—obviously 0.5 to 3.5 is a 700 percent increase, and that can only come about, in my opinion, from the ingestion of a significant amount of thallium, and that's why you have that marked increase," I said. "Thallium, by the way, is absorbed fairly rapidly, in a matter of a few hours, from the saliva into the gut, and deposits out. It takes a long time to leave the body, it has a very slow half-life and can be found many, many months after it has been ingested, especially in hair and even in other body fluids and tissues."

We went methodically through each segment and time period where the thallium level in Curley's system varied, depending on whether he most likely had been given a dose of the heavy metal or his body was excreting it and thereby lowering the concentration.

"Doctor, what is happening with regard to the thallium concentration levels in Mr. Curley's hair throughout this larger time period, that is, from June 6, 1991, through roughly September 6, 1991?" Olszewski asked.

"We see a continuous rise from June 6 down to August 31 to September 13, let's say around September 6, using a specific day," I replied. "And while there's a slight fluctuation there on July 30 to August 12, from 8 to 7.5, you see that the level is remaining high, and it gets even higher around the end of August, August 31, going into September 1, peaking out at 9.5. So during that period of time, in my opinion, Mr. Curley is ingesting repeated dosages of thallium, more than one."

I went on to explain how between the end of July and the beginning of September, Curley ingested "maintenance doses" of thallium that kept the level in his system fairly steady. The last section of the chart involved hair segments from four millimeters (or September 10) to the root, just before Curley's death. It was during this time, I testified, that Curley ingested more thallium.

"Doctor, you indicated that Mr. Curley was, in fact, a patient at the Hershey Medical Center when he was transferred there from the general hospital on September 16, through his death on September 27," Olszewski said. "What can you tell us about Mr. Curley's ingestion of thallium during that time period?"

"Well, as I've said, I do believe that he ingested one or more dosages of thallium during that time period to have gotten those significant increases," I said. "And it was during that time period, of course, that he was becoming more and more ill. He had more and more psychological problems, which, by the way, are part of the thallium toxicity picture. And it was on September 10 when alopecia, that significant hair loss, was noted. So, that all fits. The clinical, pathological, clinical toxicological correlation really is right on target."

Following the prosecutor's questions, I spent part of the afternoon being cross-examined by one of Joann Curley's defense attorneys. I returned on the second day of the hearing for more cross-examination, and her attorneys asked good questions, including ones about the validity of segmental analysis and potential thallium contamination from other sources. But there was nothing in their questioning that led me to change my opinions.

In the end, neither did the judge have a change of opinion. He ruled prosecutors presented enough evidence for the case to proceed to trial. In addition to my testimony, Justice Kane heard from Trooper Robert McBride, one of five investigators assigned to the Curley case in 1994. McBride testified that after getting forensic evidence from Dr. Rieders's hair tests, detectives spoke with Joann Curley on several occasions. They went over a list with her of people who had access to Robert Curley during at least one period when he ingested thallium. Everyone had been eliminated as a suspect except her, McBride said.

"I know what you're thinking, but I didn't kill him," Joann Curley told the detectives.

McBride also discussed a statement investigators took from a man who used to live in part of the house Robert and Joann Curley shared. The tenant described a gallon jug of rat poison that Joann Curley's grandmother gave him to deal with a rodent problem. When the man moved out in 1990, he said he left the jug in the basement. But investigators who searched the Curley house in October 1991 shortly after Robert Curley died didn't find any jug of rat poison, McBride testified.[5]

● • ●

The case against Joann Curley continued to wind its way through the courts and appeared on its way to trial. But there was an abrupt and dramatic ending on July 17, 1997, when Joann Curley appeared

289

before Judge Patrick Toole Jr. Once again, the courtroom was filled with spectators, and this time they heard Curley plead guilty to third-degree murder, admitting she killed her husband with poison. As part of the plea agreement, she gave a detailed statement to authorities. In exchange, Toole immediately sentenced her to ten to twenty years in prison.

Two days before her plea, Joann Curley sat in a second-floor conference room in the Luzerne County Correctional Facility. With her was Frank Nocito, one of her defense attorneys; two state troopers; a detective; and D.A. Olszewski. In a matter-of-fact manner, Joann Curley explained how she systematically poisoned her husband, including a final dose when he was in Hershey Medical Center because she "didn't want him to suffer anymore."

The idea to begin contaminating her husband's iced tea occurred to her when she came across the gallon-size pickle jar filled with white powdery rat poison in her basement. At that point, she said, the marriage was only several months old, but it wasn't turning out the way she thought it would. Robert Curley never hit her or even verbally abused her, she said.

"Maybe abuse is too strong a word," Joann Curley said in response to one question, "but he just wasn't like he was when we were dating. He would want things his way right then, right now."

Later in the interview, the investigators returned to questions about her motive. "If the marriage wasn't what you expected it would be and he was different than the way he had treated [you] before you got married, why not just divorce him and get rid of him?" Olszewski asked. "Why did you have to kill him?"

Her answer was chillingly succinct. "I wanted the insurance money."

For the initial poisoning, Joann Curley said she poured just a pinch of the powder into her husband's iced tea, which she mixed up in a Sunny Delight container. She said she wanted to see what it would do. The first few times, she didn't notice any difference in Robert Curley, so she said she began mixing heavier doses of rat poison into the iced tea. Even after he finally became sick in August 1991, Joann Curley said her husband continued to drink from the Sunny Delight container—which she had pushed to the back of the refrigerator so no one else would accidentally drink it. (Joann Curley said she wasn't sure how she and her daughter were exposed to thallium, and could only speculate they mistakenly drank tea from that container after Robert Curley's death. It likely wasn't a ruse after all.)

The last dose of poison came during her husband's stay at Hershey Medical Center, when she put the lethal powder in a fountain drink. She gave it to him, watched him drink some, and then left the hospital. At some point during that day, according to other court documents in the case, Robert Curley grabbed a nurse by the arm and pleaded, "Please help me. My wife is trying to kill me. She is not as she seems."

After her husband's death, Joann Curley said she threw out the Sunny Delight container and washed the contaminated thermoses, one of which Robert Curley had brought to work. She had brought tainted iced tea in the other thermos to her husband while he was in the hospital, but he never drank from it. She already had gotten rid of the large jar of rat poison several months earlier, and then disposed of a plastic bag that held a smaller amount of the deadly thallium.

When the investigation began to focus on Wilkes University and two of Robert Curley's coworkers, that suited Joann Curley just fine. And when troopers approached her in 1994 about exhuming her husband's body, she agreed because she felt doing otherwise "would be like waving a red flag." At the time, she said, she wasn't aware of the advanced testing forensic experts could do to map out a timeline of Robert Curley's thallium poisoning.

"It just never occurred to you that something like this could have been done?" Olszewski asked.

"Never," she replied. "No."

AFTERWORD

THE CASES YOU'VE JUST READ OFFER a glimpse into the power and limitations of forensic science. You've seen how forensics can help ensure that justice is served and sometimes—despite the advances of forensics—how justice can be denied.

I highly doubt Joanne Curley would have ever admitted killing her husband had it not been for the powerful evidence against her provided by the sequential hair analysis. The same holds true for the deaths in Miracle Valley. Prosecutors probably would have continued to pursue charges against the church members had it not been for the forensic evidence regarding the entrance point of bullet wounds.

Other cases showed that the "official" story may not be the most accurate. Who knows for how long Amy Grossberg and Brian

Peterson may have gone to prison had questions not been raised about the baby's grave congenital defects and about Amy's serious medical condition associated with delivery? In the case of Dr. Sam Sheppard, modern forensics was able to reach back in time and point to the most probable killer of Marilyn Sheppard. But science can do only so much. The vast preponderance of juries are composed of individuals who are dedicated to finding out the truth. However, when all is said and done, justice still is determined by men and women, who are not infallible.

Most important here, however, is that these cases have one thing in common: what initially may seem to be the obvious solution to a death may in fact be partially or completely wrong. The revelations achieved through forensic evidence can change the entire context and understanding of a crime, not to mention who did it. I hope readers enjoyed this book and perhaps learned something new. Lastly, I trust they will come away from it with a better understanding of how forensic science fits in with crime solving and within the justice system.

Cyril Wecht, M.D., J.D.

NOTES

Chapter One. Teenage Baby Killers?

1. Bernard Knight, *Forensic Pathology*, 2d ed. (New York: Oxford University Press, 1996), p. 435.

2. Transcript of *Rivera Live*, CNBC News, 18 November 1996.

3. Rich Henson, "Autopsy Shows Student's Baby Was Alive and Healthy at Birth," *Philadelphia Inquirer*, 23 November 1996.

4. Robert Hanley, "Teenagers Charged in Son's Death Return Home," *New York Times*, 1 February 1997.

5. Steve Chambers, Kelly Heyboer, and Russell Ben-Ali, "Prosecutor Awaits Autopsy in Baby Born, Killed at Prom," *Star-Ledger*, 9 June 1997.

6. Doug Most, *Always in Our Hearts* (Hackensack, N.J.: Record Books, 1999), p. 240.

Chapter Two. A Fallen Beauty Queen

1. Steve Thomas and Don Davis, *JonBenet: Inside the Ramsey Murder Investigation* (New York: St. Martin's Press, 2000), p. 14.

2. Cyril Wecht and Charles Bosworth Jr., *Who Killed JonBenet Ramsey?* (New York: Onyx, 1998), pp. 89–91.

3. Ibid., pp. 91–92.

4. Charlie Brennan, "No Need to Worry about Killer on Loose, Cops and Mayor Say," *Rocky Mountain News*, 3 January 1997.

5. Wecht and Bosworth, *Who Killed JonBenet Ramsey?* p. 99.

6. Thomas and Davis, *JonBenet*, pp. 107–108.

7. Wecht and Bosworth, *Who Killed JonBenet Ramsey?* p. 175.

8. Ibid., p. 241.

9. Thomas and Davis, *JonBenet*, p. 74.

10. Hal Haddon and Patrick Burke, letter to Alexander Hunter, Boulder County district attorney, 23 April 1997.

11. Thomas and Davis, *JonBenet*, p. 160.

12. Mary George and Ann Schrader, "Autopsy Reveals New Details," *Denver Post*, 15 July 1997.

13. Ibid.

14. Charlie Brennan, "Pathologist: No Doubt of JonBenet Sex Assault, Girl Was Hit on Head Before She Was Strangled, Expert Says," *Rocky Mountain News*, 16 July 1997.

15. Marilyn Robinson, "JonBenet Garrote Made of Paintbrush," *Denver Post*, 15 August 1997.

16. Tom Brokaw, "Former FBI Profiler Is Called in to Profile the Murderer of JonBenet Ramsey," *Dateline NBC*, 28 January 1997.

17. Wecht and Bosworth, *Who Killed JonBenet Ramsey?* p. 247.

18. Howard Pankratz, "JonBenet Knew Killer, Top Criminologist Says," *Denver Post*, 31 January 1997.

19. Thomas and Davis, *JonBenet*, p. 147.

20. Marilyn Robinson, "Ads May Influence Future Jury, Ramseys Try to Clear Name," *Denver Post*, 24 August 1997.

21. Thomas and Davis, *JonBenet*, p. 289.

22. Autopsy report from Boulder County Coroner's Office, Autopsy No. 96A-155, 27 December 1996.

23. John Ramsey and Patsy Ramsey, *The Death of Innocence: The Untold Story of JonBenet's Murder and How Its Exploitation Compro-*

mised the Pursuit of Truth (Nashville: Thomas Nelson, 2000), pp. 372–73.

24. Charlie Brennan, "Ramsey Evidence Is Explained, Hand, Boot Prints Determined to Be Innocent Occurrences," *Rocky Mountain News*, 22 August 2002.

25. Charlie Brennan, "DNA May Not Help Ramsey Inquiry; Samples Found on JonBenet's Clothing May Be from Factory," *Rocky Mountain News*, 19 November 2002.

26. Thomas and Davis, *JonBenet*, p. 306.

27. Ibid., p. 254.

28. Owen S. Good, "Ramseys Aren't Focus of Inquiry, Letter Hints," *Rocky Mountain News*, 24 December 2002.

Chapter Three. Sex, Drugs, and a Dead Casino Magnate

1. A. D. Hopkins, "Benny Binion: The Cowboy Who Pushed the Limits," *Las Vegas Review-Journal*, 2 May 1999.

2. Ibid.

3. Deposition of L. Ted Binion, Clark County, Nevada, case no. D186725, 15 February 1996, p. 31.

4. Ibid.

5. Jeff German, *Murder in Sin City* (New York: Avon Books, 2001), pp. 18, 24.

6. Glenn Puit, "Ted Binion, Troubled Gambling Figure, Dies," *Las Vegas Review-Journal*, 18 September 1998.

7. Jeff German and Jace Radke, "Former Horseshoe Exec Ted Binion Found Dead," *Las Vegas Sun*, 18 September 1998.

8. Ibid.

9. Dominick J. DiMaio and Vincent DiMaio, *Forensic Pathology*, 2d ed. (Boca Raton, Fla.: CRC Press, 2001), p. 221.

10. Peter O'Connell, "Six to Face Trial in Binion Case," *Las Vegas Review-Journal*, 14 September 1999.

11. Buddha D. Paul and Michael L. Smith, "Heroin," *Therapeutic Drug Monitoring and Toxicology* 18, no. 3 (1997): 65–74.

12. German, *Murder in Sin City*, pp. 262–63.

13. Ibid., p. 264.

14. Ibid., p. 265.

15. Bernard Knight, *Forensic Pathology*, 2d ed. (New York: Oxford University Press, 1996), pp. 358–60.

16. Ed Vogel, "Murphy, Tabish Appeals Presented," *Las Vegas Review-Journal*, 28 June 2002.

Chapter Four. The Real Fugitive

1. James Neff, *The Wrong Man: The Final Verdict on the Dr. Sam Sheppard Murder Case* (New York: Random House, 2001), p. 7.

2. Cynthia L. Cooper and Sam Reese Sheppard, *Mockery of Justice: The True Story of the Sheppard Murder Case* (Boston: Northeastern University Press, 1995), p. 51.

3. *Sheppard* v. *Maxwell*, 384 U.S. 333 (1966).

4. Neff, *The Wrong Man*, p. 91.

5. Affidavit of Paul Leland Kirk, *State of Ohio* v. *Samuel H. Sheppard*, 10 April 1955, p. 10.

6. Neff, *The Wrong Man*, p. 337.

7. Ibid., p. 341.

8. Ibid., p. 345.

9. John Affleck, "Attorneys Deliver Opening Statements in Sheppard Case," Associated Press, 14 February 2000.

10. Ibid.

11. James Ewinger and John F. Hagan, "Psychiatrist Thinks Killer Was Sadist," *Plain Dealer*, 26 February 2000.

12. Neff, *The Wrong Man*, p. 358.

13. John F. Hagan and James Ewinger, "Coroner Botched Sheppard Case, Witness Testifies," *Plain Dealer*, 29 February 2000.

14. Neff, *The Wrong Man*, p. 363.

Chapter Five. Shoot-out in Miracle Valley

1. Calvin Trillin, "Nothing but Holiness," *New Yorker*, 7 December 1981, p. 137.
2. Ibid., p. 137.
3. Ibid., p. 138.
4. "'Brother William' Finds Final Peace in the Desert," *Arizona Republic*, 24 October 1982.
5. Trillin, "Nothing but Holiness," p. 137.
6. Bud Foster, "Tragedy in Miracle Valley," KVOA-Eyewitness News 4, 12 December 1982.
7. Robert Reinhold, "Years of Tension Preceded Arizona Confrontation," *New York Times*, 25 October 1982.
8. Foster, "Tragedy in Miracle Valley."
9. Ibid.
10. "'Brother William' Finds Final Peace in the Desert."
11. Foster, "Tragedy in Miracle Valley."
12. Ibid.
13. Don Harris, "Jackson Says Church Victim of Deputies," *Arizona Republic*, 12 November 1982.
14. Foster, "Tragedy in Miracle Valley."

Chapter Six. Standing by Her Man

1. Jackie Daly, *Tammy Wynette: A Daughter Recalls Her Mother's Tragic Life and Death* (New York: G. P. Putnam's Sons, 2000), pp. 88–89.
2. Jim Patterson, "Daughter: Wynette Was Taking Narcotics and Wanted Divorce When She Died," Associated Press, 5 February 1999.
3. Bruce P. Levy, "Report of Investigation by County Medical Examiner Narrative Summary," Metropolitan Nashville and Davidson County Office of the Medical Examiner, 21 May 1999.
4. Jim Patterson, "Wynette's Body Exhumed, Autopsy Performed," Associated Press, 15 April 1999.

NOTES

Chapter Seven. The Trials of O. J.

1. Stephanie Simon, "Simpson Verdict: $25 Million; Punitive Damages Bring Total to $33.5 Million," *Los Angeles Times*, 11 February 1997.
    2. Ibid.

Chapter Eight. Robert Berdella

1. Tom Jackman, "Jury Rules in Civil Suit," *Kansas City Star*, 9 January 1992, p. A1.

Chapter Nine. Heavy Metal Murder

1. Richard Ingham, "Now It's Official: Britain Was Innocent of Napoleon's Death," *Agence France Presse*, 28 October 2002.
    2. Arthur E. Westveer, John H. Trestrail III, and Anthony Pinizzotto, "Homicidal Poisonings in the United States," *American Journal of Forensic Medicine and Pathology* 17, no. 4 (1996): 282–88.
    3. Fredric Rieders, "Report to Luzerne County District Attorney's Office," 11 March 1996, p. 4.
    4. Anthony Colarossi, "DA Tries to Derail Bail Plea," *Times Leader*, 20 December 1996.
    5. Carol Crane, "Mrs. Curley to Stand Trial," *Citizens' Voice*, 4 February 1997.

BIBLIOGRAPHY

Cooper, Cynthia L., and Sam Reese Sheppard. *Mockery of Justice: The True Story of the Sheppard Murder Case*. Boston: Northeastern University Press, 1995.

Daly, Jackie. *Tammy Wynette: A Daughter Recalls Her Mother's Tragic Life and Death*. New York: G. P. Putnam's Sons, 2000.

DiMaio, Dominick J., and Vincent DiMaio. *Forensic Pathology*. 2d ed. Boca Raton, Fla.: CRC Press, 2001.

German, Jeff. *Murder in Sin City*. New York: Avon Books, 2001.

Knight, Bernard. *Forensic Pathology*. 2d ed. New York: Oxford University Press, 1996.

Most, Doug. *Always in Our Hearts*. Hackensack, N.J.: Record Books, 1999.

Neff, James. *The Wrong Man: The Final Verdict on the Dr. Sam Sheppard Murder Case*. New York: Random House, 2001.

Ramsey, John, and Patsy Ramsey. *The Death of Innocence: The Untold Story of JonBenet's Murder and How Its Exploitation Compromised the Pursuit of Truth*. Nashville: Thomas Nelson, 2000.

BIBLIOGRAPHY

Thomas, Steve, and Don Davis. *JonBenet: Inside the Ramsey Murder Investigation*. New York: St. Martin Press, 2000.

Wecht, Cyril, and Charles Bosworth Jr. *Who Killed JonBenet Ramsey?* New York: Onyx, 1998.

Wecht, Cyril, Mark Curriden, and Benjamin Wecht. *Cause of Death: The Shocking True Stories behind the Headlines*. New York: Dutton, 1993.

———. *Grave Secrets: A Leading Forensic Expert Reveals the Startling Truth about O. J. Simpson, David Koresh, Vincent Foster, and Other Sensational Cases*. New York: Penguin, 1996.

INDEX